Our Spiritual Being Above and Beyond our Human Condition

Spirit & Form: two opposites to reconcile

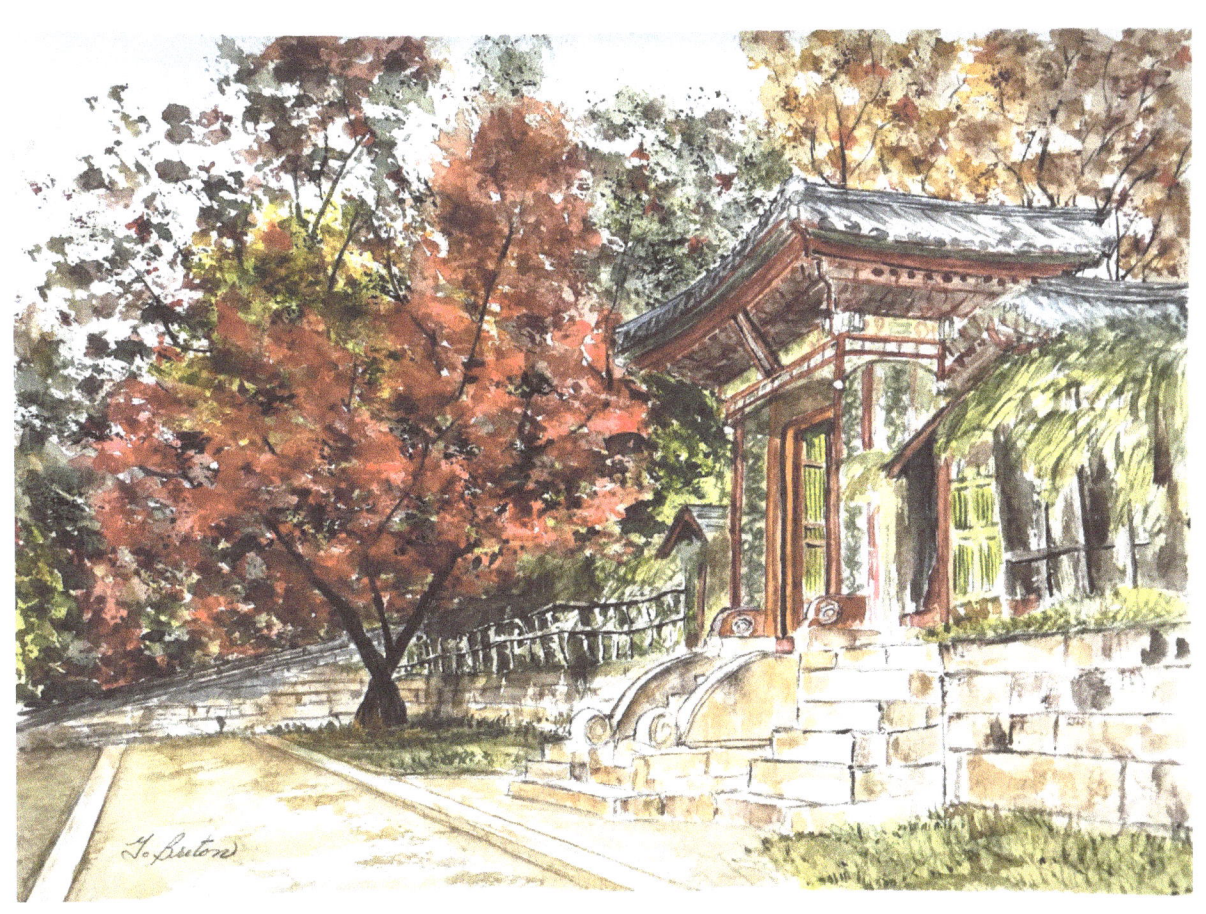

By Adrien Breton

ISBN: 979-8-89465-053-1 (sc)
ISBN: 979-8-89465-054-8(e)

Printed in the United States of America.

Integrity Publishing
39343 Harbor Hills Blvd Lady Lake,
FL 32159

www.integrity-publishing.com

Caveat – This book is for those who have started their journey on the road of discovering their spiritual being and who are not afraid of facing the nature of things, harsh as they may be. The beauty of reading a book (instead of debating ideas) is that the only arguing that can take place is with yourself. There is no place for such things as "I disagree with you," an ego-based phrase which is counterproductive in nature when looking for the truth.

Table of Contents

Becoming The Best You Can Be
as A Spiritual Being

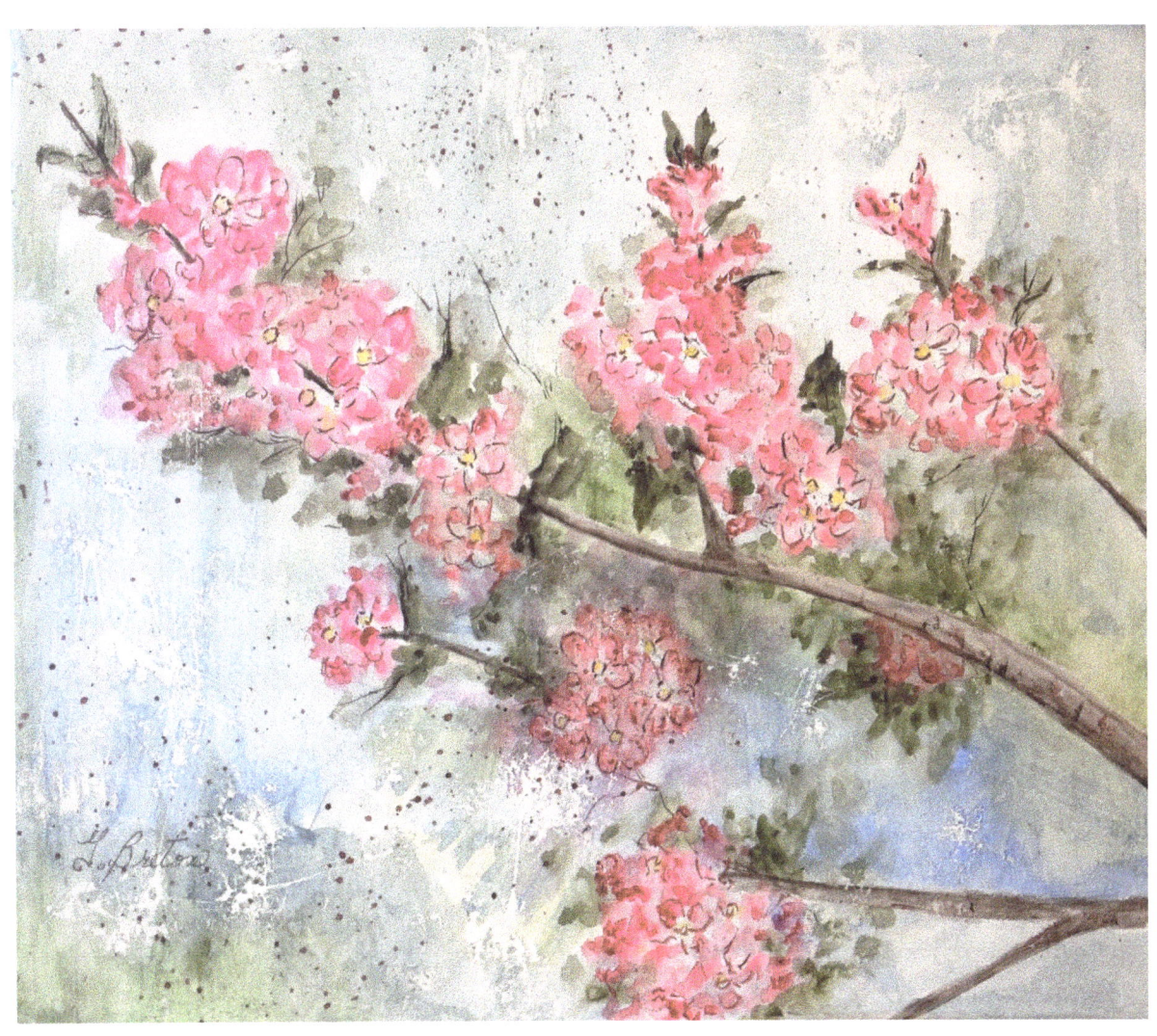

Introduction

Are We More Than Just an Evolved Animal Species?

This is a daunting question which has been addressed by innumerable thinkers from ancient times until now, long before Darwin's passage on this earth and his theory of evolution. Each philosopher proposed his or her own interpretation which, quite often, was in direct contradiction with that of a predecessor. Some, like Albert Camus professed (without affirming outright that he was an atheist) that he did not believe in God and found life to be absurd. Meanwhile, numerous religions developed over millenniums, each one having its own perception of the notion of God and of the soul of man.

I would not suggest that we all drop our daily tasks and preoccupations and plunge head on into intense meditation in order to discover our souls. For after all, we do have a physical body and share certain preoccupations with the animal kingdom, such as the need to survive. However, instead of looking for proof that we are also spiritual beings, why not simply take the time to discover our inner self? Such endless suppositions and interrogations all seem to stem from the fact that for most of us, growing up means losing contact with our inner self as the ego develops. Upon reaching adulthood, we keep wanting to compete with others (at work, in sports, and even at home). Indeed, this ego of ours must have a reason to be part of our development; but why do we all tend to further develop it and let it dominate us, dictating what we should do as it were?

In my fifty some years of teaching (languages and martial arts), I have come to realize that the most difficult obstacle to overcome when attempting to share my knowledge and experience with students, is this sense of pride attached to our domineering ego. It simply blocks or at least, hinders any appreciable learning. For me, learning is a two-way street. I constantly learn from my students and from anybody around me, including children. If the learning process is somewhat hindered in a setting where people have registered for a class, thereby implying that they are willing to learn from a person skilled in a given field, just imagine how learning is drastically blocked in everyday life, when someone expresses an opinion or makes a suggestion in a straightforward manner. "How dare you tell me what to do?" "Who does she think she is telling me to eat less fatty foods. She's not my doctor."

The only things that such a domineering ego will allow are soft, discreet suggestions. But the problem is that this approach never works. As we will see in a later chapter, in order to overcome such powerful urges such as alcoholism, bulimia, nicotine or gambling addiction, hoarding, etc.), you must reprogram your brain and completely scratch the old record with a nail, i.e., a **shock treatment**. What is this foolish idea (that we seem to entertain and strengthen) that we must PROTECT the ego? With such an attitude and this false sense of being right, no wonder we gradually lose track of our spiritual being as we grow up, thereby failing to reconcile and harmonize *spirit* and *form* ("form" being the physical world we live in, including our body).

In this book, we will look at these questions and many other considerations about the ego which systematically block our spiritual progress even before we have reached adulthood. By surmounting such obstacles blinding us to our spiritual component, we will hopefully discover that our present body is no more than a temporary vehicle for our spirit which is the actual bridge to our eternal reality.

I have used two techniques to keep us focussed on this lifelong endeavour of harmonizing with our ego: The first one is **repetition**. This will perhaps appear to some as poor writing. But again, spending almost a lifetime teaching languages and martial arts, I gradually understood and appreciated the merits of keeping focussed through repetition. The second technique is **simplicity**. It might impress some readers if I were to constantly quote the numerous authors I had the privilege to learn from and their sometimes very complex ideas. But I really came to appreciate the KISS principle often stated in one of my ju-jitsu master classes by Professor Sylvain. To paraphrase his words, I would say that it takes a long time to learn to be simple. That notion will also be looked at further on in the book.

I wish you a very profitable reading!

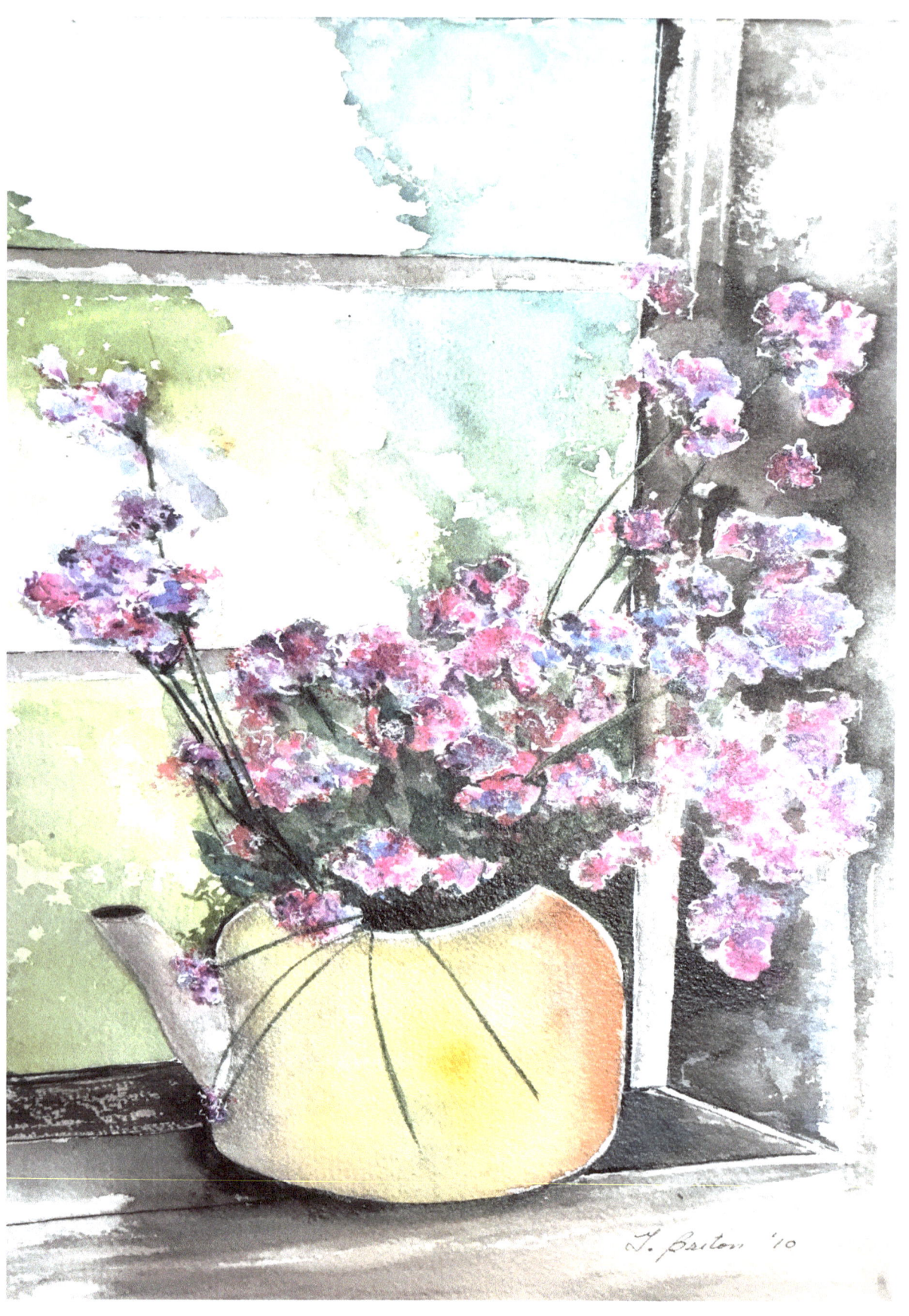

Creating Harmony Between Opposites

Is there a Dichotomy between Opposites?

You might not suspect it, but there is unbelievable power in harmonizing and reconciling opposites, contraries, or so-called "contradictions" in life (as some would view them).

In the minds of people, there exists a dichotomy between good and evil, peace and violence, light and darkness, etc. the former being supposedly desirable and the latter, condemnable. Although it may come as a surprise to many, in my opinion, this is not necessarily the case.

Huge strides were made technologically over the last century, which brought scores of "improvements" in the lives of industrialised societies. While reducing the need to count on brute force to produce any kind of staple, technology has allowed women to play a more important role and led them to demand to be treated as equals. This technology craze has permeated all walks of life and all fields of activities, be it food production or war making (as evidenced by recent televised missile launching attacks on some countries, simultaneously watched in various parts of the world as if it were a simple video game). However, such technological progress does not come without a price.

While primitive males were formerly perceived as playing an extremely important role in **sustaining life** through their ability to **kill** animals (hunting skills) or to kill invaders to protect lives in their clan (warring skills), such a natural and obvious connection between the need to kill in order to sustain life is gradually being blurred in the perception of modern inhabitants of our cities since consumers are completely disconnected from their source of meat and vegetable production. Waging wars (soldiers), chasing criminals (the police), burying the dead (undertakers), and killing animals (slaughterers), etc. are left to a minority of brave specialists while the rest of the population tries to live in a "perfect" world and has almost come to the point of thinking that their next steak or salad will come directly from the refrigerator.

Modern technology has allowed us to forget or at least, obliterate this natural interdependence between life and death. We have come to think that life can exist without death, beauty without ugliness, light without darkness, peace without war... and that the former is good while the latter is evil. But this belief is in direct contradiction with the laws of nature. There will always be fatal accidents, tidal waves, volcano irruptions, dry spells or floods, viral plagues, and all sorts of other scourges. Nature needs them to renew itself despite the strong urge of human beings to survive physically and the technological means now available to prolong life and partially erase some of the aging signs from our body. The more we alienate ourselves from our spiritual component and the more this desire to survive physically intensifies. Meanwhile, creation follows its own course and laws, no matter how much we try to oppose them in our futile attempt to perpetuate ourselves physically. Only the spiritual part of our being is meant to last beyond the boundaries of time and space. The ego tied to our material being is indeed FINITE while our spirit is INFINITE. By disconnecting ourselves from this spirit, we not only bypass the tremendous potential distinguishing us from the rest of creation, but we also violate the laws of nature in a futile attempt to make it what it wasn't meant to be.

The history of mankind alternately witnessed maternalistic and paternalistic eras. There is no doubt that, along with the emancipation of women in a western world that was increasingly becoming mechanized and now, computerized, the pendulum swung from excessive paternalistic values to the exact opposite...as it always does. Human beings, it seems, have trouble finding a balance.

Complementary Opposites

Are there absolute degrees? It might be better to speak of various degrees. For instance, although -10° C is cold, it is certainly warmer than -50° C. Even if most males have fighting qualities in their genes, developed over thousands of years, they also have some nurturing qualities to various degrees. Yet, statistics clearly show that there are at least ten times as many males as females resorting to violent means to achieve their ends, if we simply look at the number of individuals going to jail. Is anything 100% black or 100% white? There are certainly various shades in between. Hence the difficulty that most of us have to make distinctions in life. Nothing is truly black or white, despite our judicial system which demands "yes" and "no" answers without distinctions in between, so as to be more expedient. One could also say that no one is totally masculine or feminine. But things start falling into place when we create harmony between polarities.

Black is no better than white; soft is no better than hard; femininity is no better than masculinity; simplicity is no better than complexity or vice-versa. The mistake is to believe that one should be favoured over the other. Although I do not wish to minimize the sacrifices of those (Gandhi, etc.) who preached total non-violence as the only solution to the world's woes (others preached total love or more precisely, total self-negation), this seems in direct contradiction with the laws of nature since the other polarity is missing in this equation. Unfortunately, reality caught up with those who adopted this approach, and in many cases, they paid dearly when sacrificed on the altar of the implacable laws of nature. Most of them were assassinated in the process.

> Martial arts should be a way of life based on the principle of harmony between opposites rather than a simple self-defence system or method.
> *Adrien Breton*

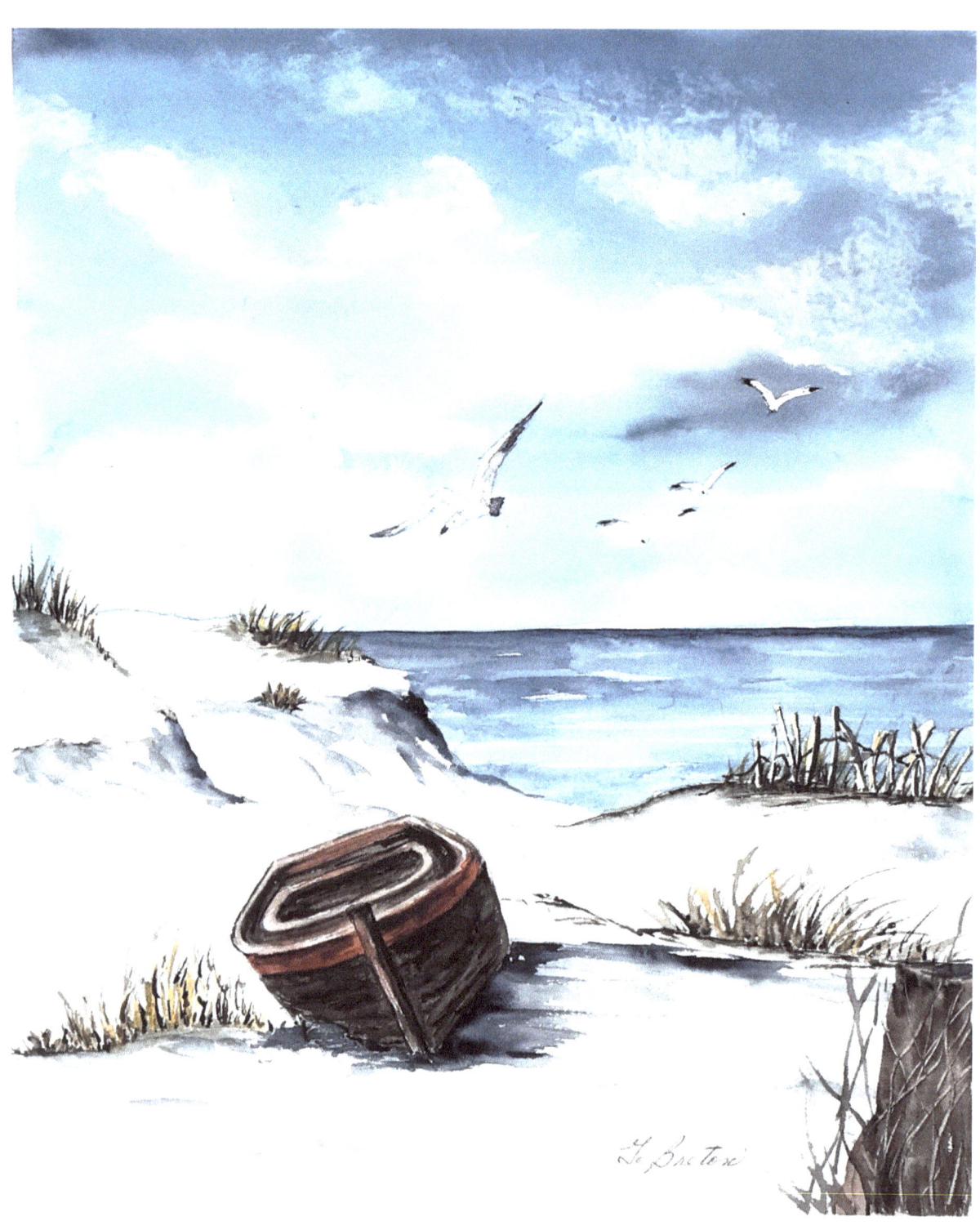

What Is Success?

> The path to success is to take massive, determined action.
> *Anthony Robbins*

Success

Success is the accomplishment of what you set out to do, step by step and day by day. It should not be measured in terms of wealth or winning (trophies, prizes, honours, etc.) For then, how much of a man or woman would you be if you measured your personal value in terms of possessions and achievements and then, an event occurred (such as an illness, a tornado, a fire, or a flood) that deprived you of what you owned? Even physical death should not part you from your true worth as an entity. Indeed, mind and body are part of the same process; they evolve from your spiritual entity which is timeless.

Apart from the gift of life, isn't freedom one of the most precious things we have and should dearly preserve? Look around you. Aren't the majority of people you know (and perhaps yourself) more than willing to sacrifice their freedom of thinking, acting and expressing themselves fully in exchange for a mere gain in materialistic comfort? Among your acquaintances, how many find profound fulfilment in what they do daily? How many are totally honest in expressing their views (tactfully, of course)? The term "politically correct" should be seen exactly for what it is namely, a "straight jacket". Is it any wonder that so many of us suffer from depression or burnout, cancer and God knows what else, since we spend most of our lives repressing our feelings and our dreams?

Humans have a need for a sense of certainty. They also seek to avoid pain at all costs. In the words of behavioural expert Dr Loretta Malandro, it is their "standard equipment". It is the way humans are wired. Yet, I believe that no true creativity can take place in the realm of the "known". In order to express our inner creativity, we must absolutely step into the "unknown" and we must also welcome the experience of "pain" (without being masochistic of course). Numerous people equate **pain** to **suffering**. But is it? If instead we look at the notion of pain as a way to grow, then where does this notion of suffering come into play? Suffering is the act of regretting the health or the wealth we used to have and lost. It is regretting the menial conditions we find ourselves in, instead of looking for solutions. Think of dire conditions such the prisoner of a Nazi concentration camp doomed to die but not resigned despite all. There are historical cases of some prisoners who never gave up and found solutions such as hiding in a pile of cadavers, waiting to be transported to a location where they would be thrown into a pit and buried. This, as it turned out, became their ticket to freedom. Resignation would have been their worst enemy, had they given up and accepted suffering as their permanent solution. In that particular case, suffering would have stemmed from a sense of helplessness. The question we might ask is "if there is hope in such extreme situations, why do most of us prefer to suffer instead when the cause of our suffering is far less dramatic than the example just given?

Part of the standard equipment of human beings is also the fundamental need "to be right" (ego). Yet, over fifty years of teaching experience have taught me that no worthwhile learning can take place in the realm of "being right". I found that learning is a two-way process and that I could learn from my students if only I set pride aside and kept an open mind. On the other hand, know-it-alls are impossible to teach to. They create little opportunity for learning. Remember that "being right" can be very costly. It can rob you of the ability to learn efficiently. Leave your ego outside your relationships and, perhaps, even outside your life.

The Pyramid

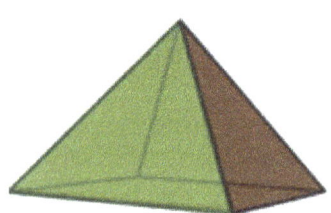

Why do the majority of people normally stay at the bottom of the pyramid instead of ascending to the apex, i.e., to unlimited possibilities? They are just very busy being right, looking for safety, and looking for pleasure while trying to avoid pain. The base or "ground level" is where the majority of people are, and this is reassuring to most people looking for safety. Being in step with the majority gives them a sense of "being right".

Consider that, as previously mentioned, for any true learning to take place you must set your pride or ego aside (stop trying to prove that you are right) and come to your teacher with a clean slate, as if you were a child (curious and coming from a position of "not knowing"). With such an attitude, "you may not look very good" but you will certainly learn much more and much faster and… it will bring you closer to your true self which is spiritual in nature.

Also, be willing to be coached by anyone, including children. While we are busy experiencing life, we tend to forget to be curious. This is a basic requirement for efficient learning.

Requirements For Overcoming the Challenges Of Life

Requirements for successful board breaking in karate	Requirements for overcoming the challenges of life	
+ Develop focus + Develop certainty + Aim beyond your target + Do not yield to pain	+ Develop focus + Develop certainty + Aim beyond your target + Do not yield to pain	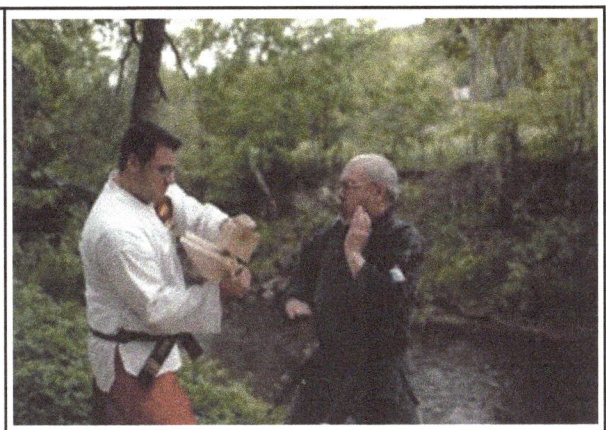

Discipline is the key to a successful life

Adrien Breton

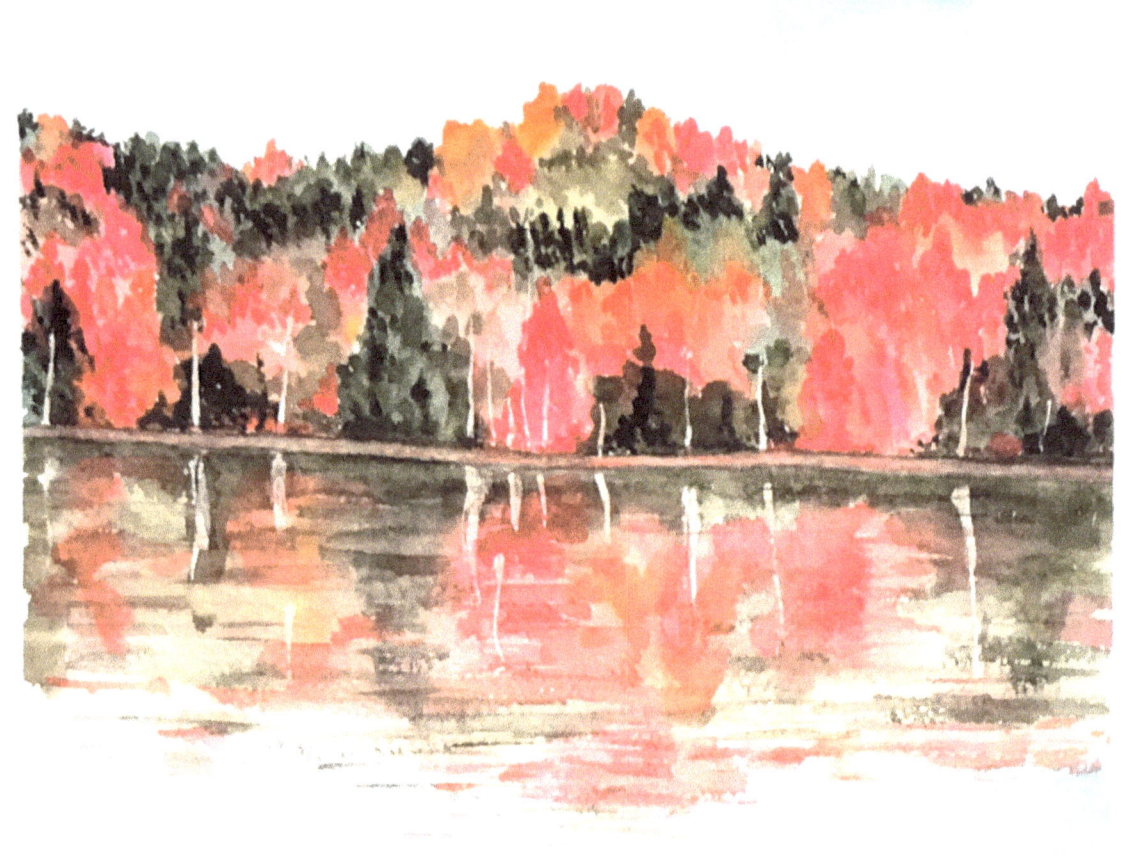

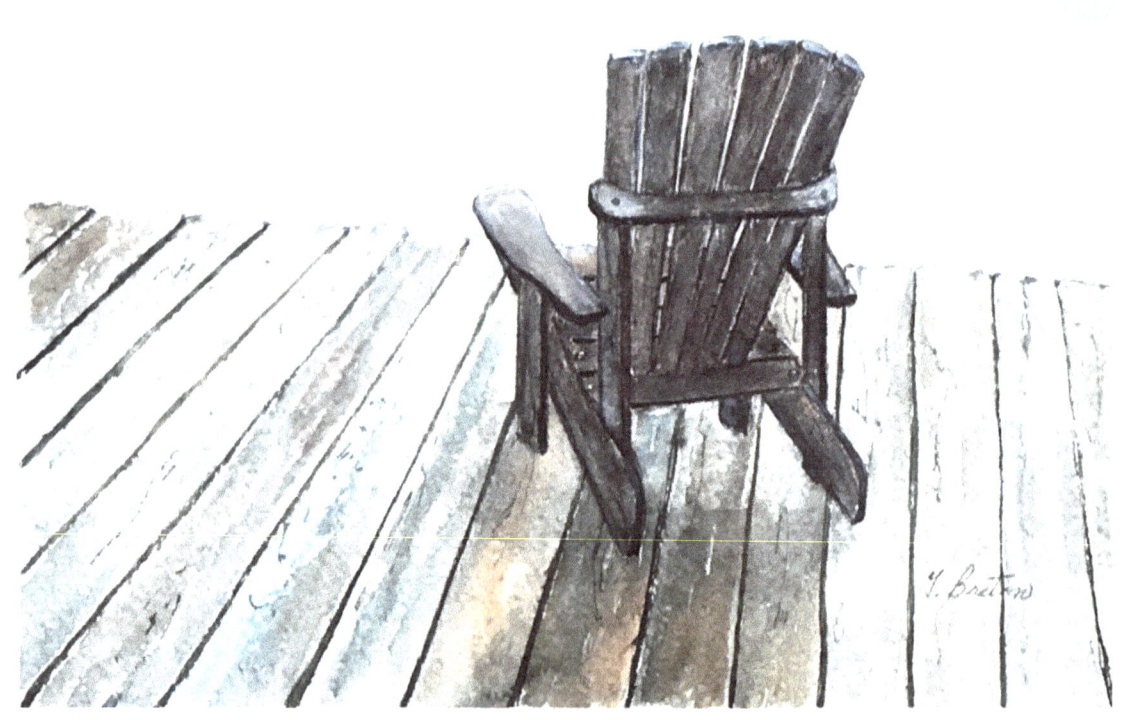

Is Violence Good or Bad? /
Debating and Arguing

Male and Female Values

Hundreds of thousands of years in the evolution of the human species have prepared males to be the best warriors and hunters possible. Now that modern evolution and the industrialisation of societies have relegated such roles to a handful of people, we are expecting males to adopt, overnight, the female values related to nurturing and cuddling.

There are various examples in nature where the male and female polarities gradually faded or fused. Life is like alternating current rather than direct current. One thing we can be sure of is that nothing stands still. Change will take place, and only you can interpret change as being for better or for worse. There is nothing basically good or bad about the notion of "nurturing" or the notion of "fighting". It is how you interpret it and what you make of it that has meaning for you and can make a difference. As a male, you can use your ingrained, programmed urge to compete (fight) to achieve positive or negative results. "Positive" and "negative" are neither "good" nor "bad". It depends on the interpretation given to it by you and the members of the society you live in.

For instance, in some former cultures, some say (although it has never been confirmed) that it was considered desirable i.e., "good" to destroy infants who came into the world with inborn deficiencies by throwing them over a cliff. Right now, this notion is considered as horrendous by most. Yet, the option of destroying a perfectly healthy baby in its mother's womb is not only considered good and acceptable to a great number of people in our society, but it is also legal in many countries. I personally do not pass judgement on what is considered "good" or "bad" by any given society at any given time in the history of mankind and prefer to let prevailing laws dictate what is acceptable or not for the majority. For, the debate about the mother's freedom of choice as opposed to the elimination of an embryo or fetus can only be settled through "majority rule" according to predominant values in a given society.

Following the horrors of the two world wars and the ensuing industrialization, a good part of the human race almost universally united in adopting "nurturing" values to the detriment of "fighting" values. Yet, look at the way we treat victims of crimes today. Criminals enjoy much better protection and support than victims do. Nature is being assaulted from all fronts by our constant modernisation endeavours. We destroy our wildlife and our forests, we pollute our oceans and streams but also, the air we breathe, all in the name of progress. This may go on to the point of extinction if we don't mend our ways.

Did you ever stop to think about the carnage taking place on our roads? Since there is a consensus among the members of modern society that we will not dispense with vehicles, dismembering people in traffic accidents seems to be acceptable (although no one will admit to it – but reality speaks louder than words) ... until it happens to your own family or friends, of course. Yet, it was quite predictable that there would be casualties involved when thousands of vehicles crisscross each other on roads and highways at higher velocities than walking speed. Here, the laws of nature are at work as always, and they take precedence over the laws of the human species. We are quite ridiculous in the way we violate the laws of nature and then act very surprised when "accidents" occur. But, as always, when a majority of people think or act in a particular way, the rest of society follows in their footsteps thinking that this must be the right way since majority rules.

Debating and Arguing

Just as "competition" is the drive that fuels most human endeavours, even though the ego may not be the best fuel for accomplishing anything worthwhile, "debating/arguing" also ranks first as to the way to communicate and share ideas with others. Again, pride and the ego are at work here. It is part of the standard equipment of human beings to want to prove they are right. Even when performed in the most civilized of manners, debates are a complete waste of time and energy in my view, and they are also destructive in many ways. Again, the forces at work in a debate are the desire to prove that one's opinion is better than the other person's.

We all intrinsically know what is best i.e., what is in harmony with nature (what most religions call "conscience".) We simply keep blurring the image so as to make it fit our immediate interest according to the choices we have made so far in life. As you read these lines, you are perfectly free to adopt or reject any of the ideas expressed by the author. Where is the need for debate? If you don't agree with any or all ideas contained herein, simply don't make them yours… I am sharing my perception of life as my own experience and previous choices dictate it. But your experience of life may be quite different from mine, which is OK. There is absolutely no need to argue about anything. **Sharing** your views is one thing, but **debating and arguing** is quite different. On the other hand, the only things truly worth fighting for, it seems to me, are the protection of the gift of life and freedom of choice. In other words, I would personally be prepared to fight only to protect life and liberty.

If you stop competing, if you stop arguing and debating, the whole picture about creation and what you are fundamentally becomes much clearer. You then have a better chance of starting to look for harmony between opposites. In doing so, you are beginning to bring your worst enemy under control namely, yourself.

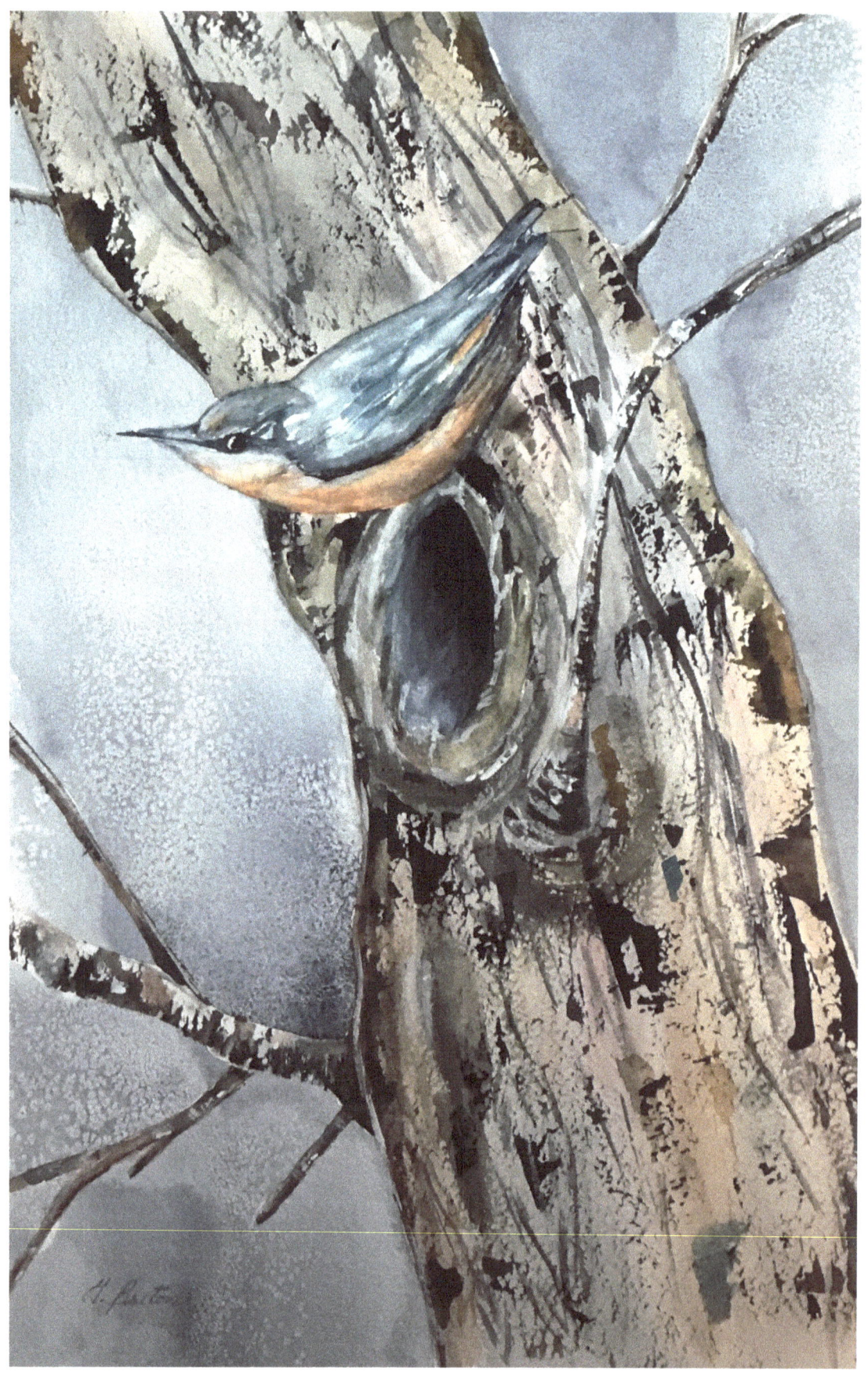

Pain Is Your Ally /
Repetition Is the Mother of Skill /
The Importance of Making Distinctions /
It Is Easy to Love Loveable People /
Contradictory Expectations

It is a natural instinct for people to try to avoid pain at all costs and to look for pleasure in everything. Far from me is the idea of suggesting that we should delight in pain as masochists do. It is quite natural to look for pleasure and to try to avoid pain. In fact, it is the way that humans are wired. Yet, here again, we should strive to achieve balance between pain and pleasure. Such is our challenge as human beings. Pain serves a very useful role in many situations. For instance, physical pain may serve as a warning signal that something is going askew. Painful experiences may tell us that it is time to change certain choices in our lives. Even pain which appears to us as completely purposeless may have a hidden agenda. We must learn to trust destiny. Pain can be our ally if we learn from it. What we actually perceive as short-term pain may in fact lead to long-term pleasure. Many people live ordinary lives of resignation because they respond to pain negatively and try to avoid it at all costs. Here again, we must learn the value of a balanced approach between pain and pleasure. All of this is not a matter of resignation but rather of mastery of the self. And remember, as previously mentioned, that the notion of **pain** should not be confused with that of **suffering**.

Repetition Is the Mother Of Skill

Repeating certain gestures, moves, or sounds (in painting, music, language learning, sports, etc.) over the course of a lifetime may seem boring to some. However, no true mastery can come about without constant repetition. Every master knows that. The problem is that one tends to look for short-term results in an attempt to "save steps" and still look as an expert. So, we use shortcuts. If the course you trace for yourself is one where the ego takes a backseat and long-term results are built upon the enjoyment of the present or here-and-now, you will find great pleasure in repetition.

The Importance of Making Distinctions

Learn to make distinctions between actual events and your interpretation of them. If your quest is to avoid pain at all costs, you may end up interpreting challenging events as something quite undesirable. Since avoiding pain and looking for pleasure is part of the standard equipment of human beings, only those who learn to give empowering interpretations to all human experiences can hope to make a major difference in their lives. Why is it that losing someone dear to us is seen as undesirable by most while a few exceptional individuals use such an event as a springboard to go beyond their present abilities? We could ask the same question about those who become paraplegic in a car accident, etc. Your interpretation of events is what makes a difference... not the event itself, no matter how painful it was.

When someone is battling with a serious illness or gets seriously injured in a car accident, the very first question that comes to mind is "why me?" All of a sudden, all the precious moments we enjoyed so far in our life, the many talents we have, the undeserved quality of services we enjoy in our country, and God knows what else, no longer count. Our sole interpretation of the event we are confronted with is a negative and disempowering one. "Why me?" Instead, could we not make important distinctions and wonder what this new challenge will teach us and how it will make us better people if we face it head on? Our problem is not that we had bad luck but rather that we fail to make proper distinctions; we fail to develop an empowering interpretation of the event. It is not what we receive from life that makes any difference but rather, what we make of what we've received.

> To get better results, you need better questions.
> "Why me?" is not a very useful question.
> *Adrien Breton*

It Is Easy to Love Loveable People

Isn't it easy to love lovable people? Everybody does! You come across a sweet person who only has compliments for you and you immediately feel sympathy for this individual. Again, your ego is at work here. It is so easy to lap up all this attention. But how much do you learn from someone who never confronts you and always "dances to your tune?"

Far more difficult is the task of loving those who envy you, begrudge you for your accomplishments, and criticize you without reason. Showing love and compassion to these people may not be as easy, but it is a great opportunity to deflate the ego and become a better person in the process. In conclusion, when your ego tries to "protect" you and you listen to it, you are losing a great opportunity to become wiser as you grow older. Since most people cater to their ego first and foremost and since we strive to avoid pain at all cost, no wonder so many become grouchy individuals as they advance in years. View such individuals as an empowering tool to constantly evolve into a better person until your very last breath.

Contradictory Expectations – Food for Thought

When politicians express their true feelings and thoughts, every movement and organization representing minorities, etc. get on their case. As a result, they start using stereotypes and a set language. Then, the public at large blame them for never speaking candidly. Such are life's contradictions that need to be reconciled and harmonized.

True Friends

We expect true friends to be candid with us and tell us what they think. Yet, when they do, don't we react by rejecting them instead of showing appreciation for the opportunity they are giving us to truly look at ourselves and improve? Why does our ego take over and feels the need to "protect" us against such rare individuals who are willing to take risks because they truly care for us? Do we really want to be surrounded with Facebook friends and "sympathizers" instead of truly caring and honest people? Here again, we seem to have contradictory expectations and disempowering interpretations.

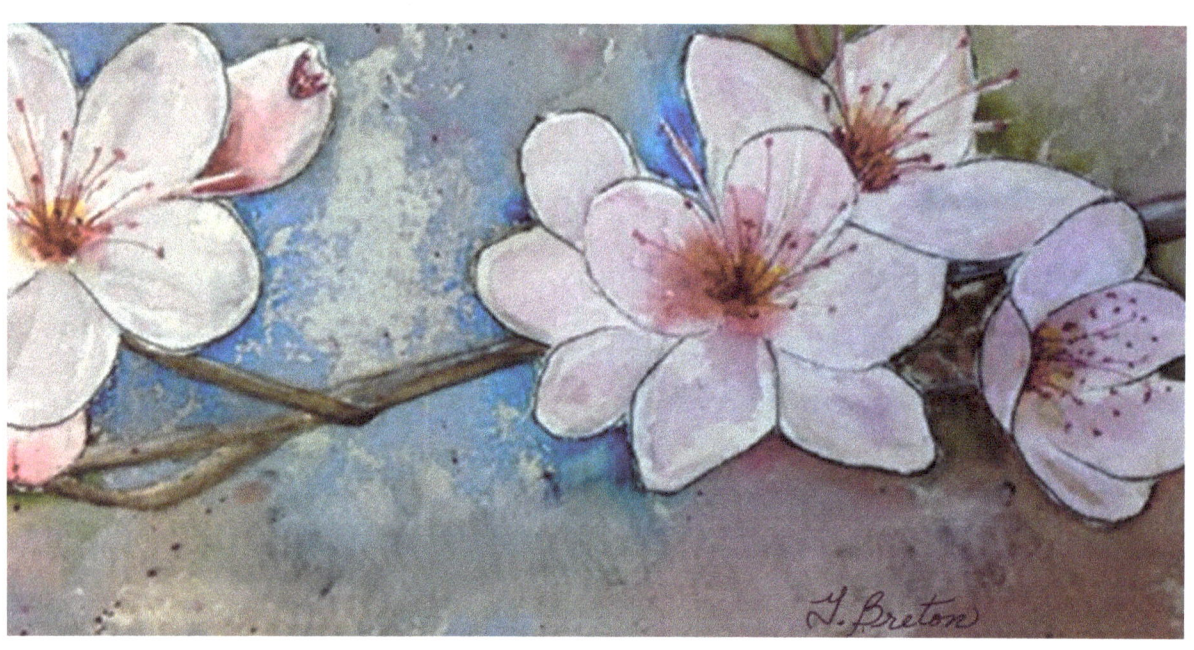

Simplicity Versus Complexity /
Is The Universe Simple or Complex? /
One's Perception of The World Is
Based on One's Experience

Simplicity Versus Complexity

"It takes a long time to learn to be simple." What this statement implies, though, is that one first has to evolve towards complexity. This is true of learning a profession such as translation, medicine, or any other complex professional activity. There is a huge difference between being simple and being simplistic.

Human growth allows no shortcut. Every step counts in coming full circle to reach maturity. Think of the development stage of a child who now knows how to stand up and walk erect. From then on, there is a long journey (lifetime) ahead for him. Mastering the guitar or the keyboard is yet another good example. One can learn fairly quickly to play basic chords and their minor and major variations in order to strum a tune and sing along. But it doesn't make you a master in music. It is quite legitimate to decide not to become a true master in any given field of expertise. It is another thing, however, to maintain the illusion and believe that you have mastered the said art and set yourself up as an example for others to follow. Humility and honesty should always play a role in the state of not knowing. "Growing humble" is also part of this life-long process. It is part of conquering the ego.

Is the Universe Simple or Complex?

For some earlier thinkers such as Aristotle, there were only four basic elements namely, fire, earth, air, and water. Yet, modern science keeps adding chemical elements to its periodic table as new discoveries are being made. Increasingly powerful telescopes allow us to discover new galaxies billions of light years away. The complexity and immensity of the universe is still beyond man's grasp. Is this to say that the universe is indeed complex?

Not really, if we succeed in reconciling such notions as "time" and "timeless," "space" and "spaceless." Creation is both simple and complex depending on your perception of it which, in turn, depends on your experience of life and the world around you. A young child experiences gravity by dropping objects onto the floor. He discovers his body by touching it. For his current development, this simple approach is all that is required to make him fully functional. However, in order to become a lifesaving surgeon, this young human being has a long way to go into the complexities of the human body. I have had the privilege to read some authors whose technical knowledge of the universe is astounding. For instance, I recently finished listening to Stephen Hawking's audio book titled *The Grand Design* (written in collaboration with Leanard Mlodinow). Hawking's knowledge of quantum mechanics and of Einstein's theory of relativity is so profound that I would be at a loss to master even half of his book's content on the subject. Yet, although he repeatedly refers to Einstein and the impact his theory had on modern science, he seems not to share Einstein's belief in a supreme being. (Einstein was recorded as saying that "God does not play dice with the Universe," among such numerous clues of his perception on this matter.) Many well-known authors such as Deepak Chopra tell us to look within ourselves to find the divine. Doctor Chopra's and such other authors' knowledge of the universe is also quite impressive. But he shares with us the simple step of looking into ourselves to discover the truth about divinity, which no amount of knowledge of the universe is able to reveal. The real challenge for us as we grow wiser is to create harmony between simplicity and complexity, never losing track of the role each has to play. There is really nothing so complex about discovering our spiritual being; the real task, however, is to conquer both our ego and the notion of *duality* which pits so-called opposites one against the other instead of harmonizing them. There lies the real challenge.

One's Perception of the World Is Based On One's Experience.

The snowed-in driveway – I used to have a driveway which was approximately 150 feet (45 m) deep to which a two-car parking lot was attached on the side. In the wintertime, when a snowstorm would hit this Quebec region where my house was located and the snow was drifting, it used to take me a solid three hours or more to clear it with the help of my snow scoop before I finally could afford to buy a snow blower. My next-door neighbour's house was located much closer to the street and, in addition to not having a two-car parking lot to clear, her driveway measured approximately 50 feet (15 m) in depth. One winter day, as I had been shovelling for over two hours and the job was far from being over, she came out with her shovel and upon seeing me she greeted me and shouted: "Did you notice how much more snow I have to clear than you do? This drifting snow seems to pile up much more in my driveway than yours." Half an hour later, I was still at it and she was back in the house, her driveway completely cleared. Do you get the point? She hated shovelling so much that to her, mother nature was not being fair and piled up the snow much more in her driveway than in anybody else's. This perception of hers could have easily been challenged with a simple measuring tape, but I'm sure she would have kept on believing that her task of clearing the snow was far greater than mine. So, I just kept on shovelling without arguing in order to keep the peace and avoid useless arguments.

The car make – Although you had always been driving around in a real gas guzzler, you eventually got tired of the price of petrol constantly reaching new heights and were now ready to listen to arguments about the virtues of small economical models. One day, a friend of yours bragged about his new acquisition and about how much he was now saving since he had purchased his new Yaris. You had never noticed this car make before or heard of it but trusted your neighbour and rushed out to buy one since your old clunker was about to give up on you anyway. A few days later, while proudly driving your brand-new small Yaris, you told your wife: "Did you notice honey how popular the Yaris is? There seems to be one passing by every few minutes. Now that YOU had experienced the reality of a Yaris, you were able to see them (which had not been the case so far).

The chronic couch potato – Who doesn't know someone (a family member or otherwise) who spends most of his time watching life unfold on TV or the screen while exerting very little physical effort, apart from getting up to go to the fridge, when not delegating that task to a spouse? Yet, you don't need to spend too much time in the company of such individuals to find out that they have quite strong and set opinions about everyone, particularly those who are very busy trying to make a difference for society such as politicians or other similar professionals. Since their life is mostly based on watching rather than taking action, they run very little risk of making mistakes, but have plenty of time to criticize those who do.

Unions versus business entrepreneurs are another case in point – If we were to look at the labour world simplistically, we could group entrepreneurs on one side and union workers on the other. Entrepreneurs soon find out that in order not to be part of statistics showing most of them as going bankrupt during the first few years and losing their shirts, houses, etc. in the process, they have to work extremely long hours (70 hours or more a week) for many years and accept earning far less than their employees. A few ingenuous and persevering ones eventually make it after having sacrificed their marriage, their house and sometimes their health in the process. It is at this stage that their employees start talking about forming a union in order to get their "fair share" of the profits. On the other hand, the unionized worker may feel that he has given the best years of his life serving the interests of his employers. It may then be hard to understand if, one day, the company brings its operations to a close and lays everybody off on short notice.

Such is human nature; we truly perceive things only once we have experienced them ourselves. Prior to that, in a manner of speaking, they do not exist for us. No wonder people can argue for hours on end in disagreement. Hence the need for humility, faith, trust, acceptance, and open-mindedness. Only through developing such qualities can we hope to make use of other people's experience and progress much faster in life. If you are convinced that you are the sole guardian of the truth, chances are you will die a stubborn, narrow-minded old man after years of arguing uselessly.

As I have tried to illustrate with the previous cases, your perception of the world is directly influenced by the way you experience it. This is why I strongly urge anyone to take up a traditional martial art, especially one that excludes the notion of competition and stresses harmony between opposites… one that is all-encompassing and balanced, not focussing on a given, specialized aspect. Such a vehicle for harmonious development between body and mind will make you experience life in all its so-called contradictions and lead you to personal fulfilment and, hopefully, to spiritual development.

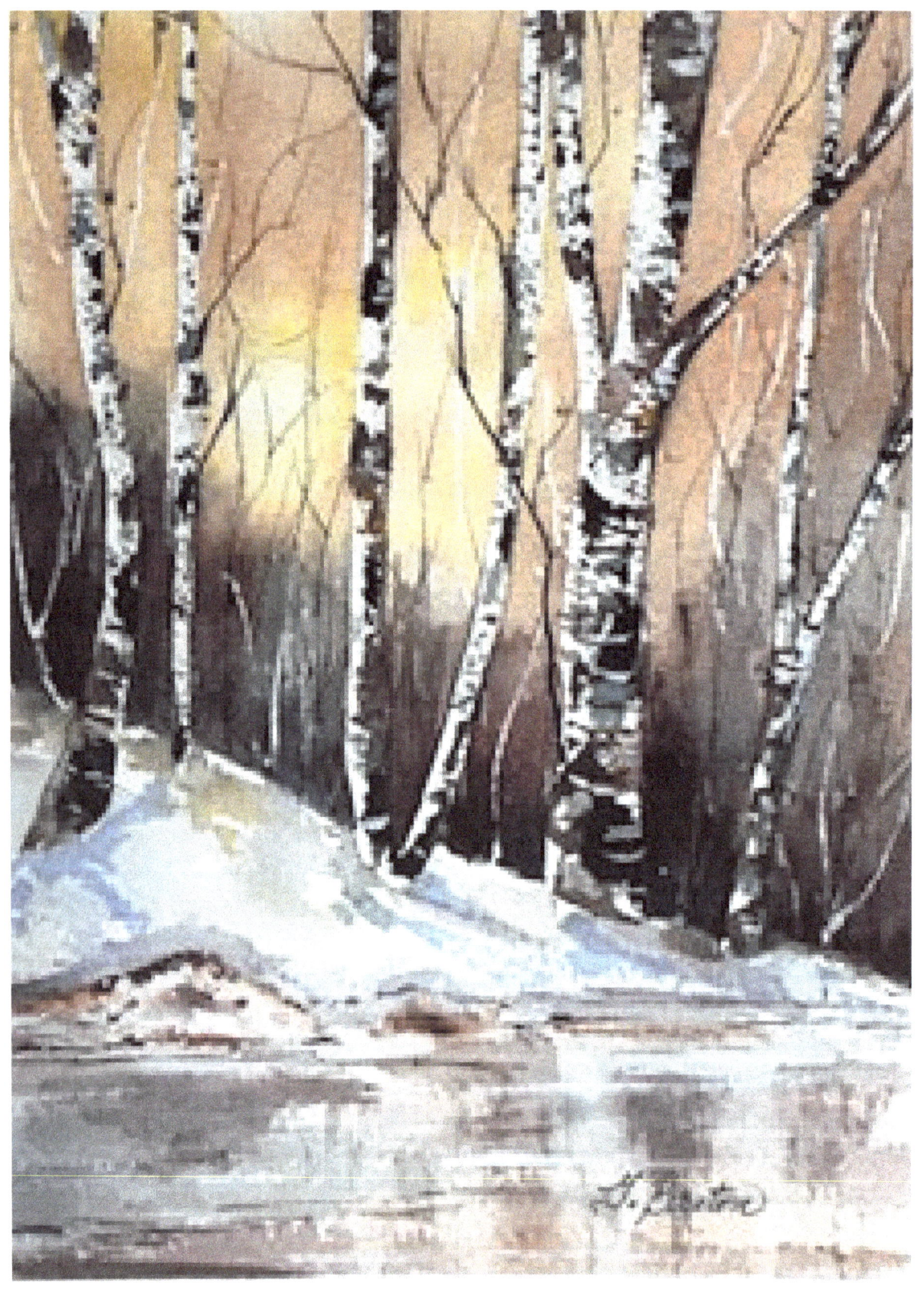

An Alert Mind /
Our Values /
The Samurai Code of Honour /
Do We Own Anything?

An Alert Mind (Which The Japanese Call "Zanshin")

The best way to face the various challenges of life is to keep an alert mind at all times i.e., to let the mind free to react to any given circumstances and free of any inhibiting thoughts or prejudices.

In everyday situations, the mind can be imprisoned by preconceived ideas and prejudices. Some people feel that they have to have an opinion about everything and everyone. They find safety and comfort in *judging* others and placing them in pre-set categories where such "victims" of their *judgment* are given no chance of escape. This approach to others may initially provide a false sense of safety but eventually, it is bound to stifle creativity and harmony. How can anybody have a chance to impact your life if the only contributions you accept from them are those that "fit" your preconceived ideas and prejudices? Keep an open mind and stay alert; **practice zanshin.** By being different from you and expressing divergent views, people pause no threat to you whatsoever, unless your whole life's foundations stand on shaky grounds… in which case I would suggest reconstructing your foundations from scratch on more solid grounds. For, a house with shaky foundations stands absolutely no chance of ever withstanding the inevitable storms nature has in store for us.

> How can you influence somebody's life positively
> if you are judging that person?
> *Adrien Breton*

23

The pitfall with prejudices is that, in many cases, they are founded. Let us take *age* for instance. At the time of writing this paragraph, I am 77 years old and there is a definite shortage of labour in many countries, including Canada. For instance, in the case of teaching languages (which is one of my occupations), there has even been discussions about accepting people of lesser experience and training in public schools and the public sector in order to counter this shortage. So, for a while now, I have "tested the waters" on a few occasions and applied for part-time positions, but to no avail. *Silence* is normally the weapon used by those in charge of selecting applicants, since age discrimination is forbidden by law. You might think that the quality of services would be the primary goal of such organizations… but is it? Then, you might also think that one of the other preoccupations could be the number of years you would stay in someone's employ. Yet, a quick glance at the number of years a young person would presently (year 2024) stay in one particular job would reveal that job mobility has never been so high and that most new employees are quick to jump on new and better paid opportunities. For a great number of them, a few years may be what you can best hope for. Chances are that someone my age would last longer. I could go on mentioning other aspects such as adaptability to new technologies, etc. Now, if someone with well over fifty years experience and a very solid background in teaching languages at the university and college levels is being "ignored," then the question is: Isn't that a clear case of age discrimination? Of course, it is; but unfortunately, the prejudice is well founded. I have come across all types of people in all walks of life who dream about retiring at age 60 or even less. As they grow older, an overwhelming proportion of them lose their drive, passion, and flexibility as they increasingly become sedentary. So, should we conclude that our well-founded prejudices are useful in selecting candidates? The answer is yes, if you are **NOT** truly looking for the most competent, stable, passionate, and dedicated candidates. Why? Just think for a moment! If someone makes it to 70 or more with a far superior baggage of experience, wisdom, knowledge, flexibility, passion, dedication, etc., chances are that you are simply bypassing an opportunity to chose among a small minority of exceptional candidates. As I write these lines, the French classical pianist Colette Maze comes to mind. At age 109, she released her last album in 2023 prior to her death. Listen to it and again, ask yourself if the prejudice against age is a good selection criteria when one is truly looking for excellence. Prejudices, no matter what category of people are involved, are the easy and quick selection tools chosen by the majority who is satisfied with mediocre results. If prejudices guide you, you are the actual loser; not the person you offhandedly ignored. Keep an alert mind (ZANSHIN) instead of opting for quick and easy solutions. My wish is for all of us to become the best we can be. For, this is our destiny.

Our Values / The Samurai Code of Honour

Over the centuries, the samurai developed a Code of honour known as Bushido which guided many of his actions. One of his many duties was loyalty to his Daimyo. Should he dishonour his lord through his actions, the samurai was expected to commit seppuku or suicide by ripping his stomach open i.e., by way of disembowelment. Talk about a "drastic" and violent action! Many other radical actions of the samurai were dictated by this code.

Similarly (as we grow up), we develop values which guide our actions throughout our entire life. Some are inherited from society or laws governing us (such as the obligation not to kill our fellow man) while others take shape on the basis of our personal experiences (such as the way we respond to verbal or physical attacks). There may be times when our personal values are in direct conflict with the values of society. For instance, if I grew up in an environment where I had to replace family members with members of a clan (criminal gang or otherwise) in order to develop a sense of belonging, I may have inherited a code of conduct dictating that I harm or kill someone in order to go up the ranks and prove myself to others in the clan.

But whatever our past experiences dictate, we should remember that, through our spiritual being, we are basically free to decide what values to adopt. Therefore, if you wish to live in harmony with the rest of society, be careful of the values you adopt and adapt them if need be; for, they will indeed dictate how you behave under stress (and even, in your daily lives) as surely as the Bushido dictated the samurai's behaviour.

One of the basic ingredients sadly lacking from most people's behaviour is that of COURAGE. Yet, it takes much courage from the samurai in you to "reprogram" your brain with shock treatment to drop certain destructive habits or patterns from your life. A good example of this is that of smoking. How many people do you know tried the "soft" approach such as patches, kind reminders from friends, etc. only to fall right back into the same groove and pick up smoking again? On the other hand, how much suffering is attached to overeating? People look for miraculous solutions and diets instead of showing courage. If, the next time you catch yourself eating fatty foods or overeating in a restaurant, you were to stand up on your chair and shout out loud to everyone around "look at the pig I am" while pointing at your plate, I am pretty sure that your misery would be over and that you would never overeat again. This type of example has been given time and time again by NLP (neurolinguistic programming) specialists. It definitely works since it stops you dead in your tracks (drastic measure) and reprograms your brain so that you may make new, healthier choices. Yet, whether they admit it or not, in an attempt to spare their ego, most people would rather go on suffering for the rest of their life instead of taking this or other kinds of drastic measures to solve a major problem once and for all.

How many times have I personally been considered "lucky" by people learning that I had stopped smoking or that I went from being an almost hopeless alcoholic to a moderate drinker, etc.? When learning about such feats, friends will ask for your advice or even assistance. But beware! Most are looking for "soft" and "quick" solutions and will reject YOU if you bring them the "drastic" solution, even though they were the ones telling you about their problem initially. You will soon find out that their ego is far more important than anything else, including their health and your friendship.

Sparing the ego is just about universal and is expressed in many ways… not just through sheer pride. For instance, in a language learning situation, a student may tell you that she is shy to express herself before the group. "They all seem to be much better than I am," she will say. In a personal relationship, a person may say that being sensitive in nature, he was deeply hurt by his friend's comments regarding his appearance. Being shy, hurt, insulted, etc. is all part of sparing the ego. If you want to really make a difference in your life, be humble, candid, and open. Hear what the other person is saying instead of immediately rejecting what was said. Who knows? You might discover some truth in it, which will help you change for the better. The only time you should discard this friend's words is if there is an obvious attempt at diminishing you. Remember this obvious truth: no one can really hurt your feelings unless you let them do so. If they behave that way, simply remember that they still have a long way to go and may need assistance in becoming better persons; rejecting them would certainly not fulfil this objective. As stated elsewhere in this book, it is easy to love lovable people. Everybody does! Through fear, the need for safety, etc., the majority of people normally stay at the bottom of the pyramid instead of ascending to the apex. You will discover the "grandeur" of your soul if you do not let an overbearing ego dominate you. Make it your ally instead.

Do We Own Anything? Do We "Own" Our Children for That Matter?

> Your children are not your children. They are the sons and daughters of Life's longing for itself. They come through you but not from you; and though they are with you, yet they belong not to you.
> *Kahlil Gibran*

Looking at the way people behave with their children, you would think they "own" them. How many parents treat their children as if they were their possession? This is particularly true in the twenty-first century that has seen quite a few parents abdicate their role as educators. We are indeed far from some "primitive" clans where all members of a given collectivity were involved in raising all children. Couples are so busy working outside the home pursuing a career that the home has become an empty nest and there is no one to look after the education of these latchkey children when they return from school. Worst still, although you might expect such "absenteeism" in parenthood to lead to the delegation of the disciplinary tasks (be it to school teachers, educators, and guardians), the exact opposite is taking place. Educators are constantly being hindered by the parents themselves in their task of disciplining the children entrusted to their care.

It may be that, out of a sense of guilt or other such motives, abdicating parents think that opposing a detention imposed on their misbehaving child will endear them to their forsaken offspring. And to gain this undeserved appreciation, they go as far as bribing their children with excessive material possessions as if this could ever earn them the respect they do not deserve by abdicating their role as educators.

If you were inspired by the collective effort of raising children in a clan, just try scolding a rowdy little brat in a public place. You'll see how quickly the parents who had been completely ignoring their misbehaving child so far will come to his "rescue" and get on your case. How dare you discipline "their" dear little jerk … their "possession"? No wonder there is no sense of community and of the common good anymore! And of course, we make sure our laws are amended to comply with this behaviour. At the moment of writing these lines, the Criminal Code of Canada still states that "Every schoolteacher, parent or person standing in the place of a parent is justified in using force by way of correction toward a pupil or child, as the case may be, who is under his care, if the force does not exceed what is reasonable under the circumstances." But there are lobbyists working very hard here at home as well as in Europe to make sure such "barbaric" laws are amended as soon as possible. It would never occur to these people to look at how nature handles such cases (the lioness with her cubs, for instance). After all, we are much more evolved than these animals, aren't we? No matter how "domesticated" and civilized human beings become, they will always be guided by the basic animal instinct of protecting themselves against dangerous and violent individuals (and yes… there are unbalanced teenagers and children as well who can be extremely violent). You may wish to perceive yourself as very different from mother lion who strikes her cub with her paw to protect it against a looming danger; but are you really?

If some people can go on living in dreamland, it is because in a civilized society, they are protected by an army, a police force, etc. doing the dirty work for them. When a majority of do-gooders unaware of the realities of criminal or delinquent minds participate in lobbies to change the laws for the majority, they unwillingly protect criminals, which leads to a complete unbalance between the rights of criminals and those of law-abiding citizens. We end up seeing the victims of crime being afforded much less support than those who assaulted them. Worse still, with such biased laws, the victim of an aggression can end up being victimized a second time by the legal system because he or she had the "misfortune" of defending himself or herself successfully against an aggressor.

In such cases, I suggest abiding first and foremost by the laws of nature. You stand a much better chance of protecting your life and that of your loved ones, should you ever be aggressed wildly by a person out of control. Rather than ending up dismembered or at the morgue, I would prefer to be still alive and capable of standing before a court judge who will then send me to jail on the false premise that there is such a thing as the "use of excessive force" when being faced with a deadly threat. If someone decides to put my life in danger, I do not abide by the modern legal notion that I should take out a measuring tape to assess the force continuum and run even the slightest risk of being killed for a decision made by the aggressor himself.

No one needs to share the above view. But those who do may find a solution in creating harmony between mind and body, violence and peace, and so forth rather than ignoring one polarity under the false assumption that one can exist without the other. Nature will always stand guard to redress the balance no matter what laws are adopted by any given society.

I do not "own" my children any more than I "own" my life; but I am the "guardian" of that gift and it is my very first and basic duty to protect it, no matter how misguided human beings may be in passing unfair and unreasonable laws. It is my strongest hope to live in peace and harmony with the animal kingdom and with my fellow human beings. However, anyone taking it upon himself to threaten my life will not be given any chance to succeed despite unfair laws protecting him to the detriment of law-abiding citizens. By perceiving human nature the way it is instead of the way I wish it were, I stand a much better chance of reaching true harmony with the rest of creation.

You would be well advised to develop COURAGE and HUMILITY in order to solve your recurring problems once and for all. The next time you are faced with a gruelling decision about a major flaw in your life, remember the Samurai Code of Honour and show COURAGE. This is the only "miracle solution." If ever you are lucky enough to have a courageous but foolish friend telling you that you "stink" (shock treatment vocabulary to help you reprogram your brain) because of your smoking habit, do not reject him to protect your ego… Instead, take responsibility, show COURAGE and HUMILITY, and accept the "drastic comment." It may very well be the push you needed to reprogram your brain and stop smoking once and for all. The price to pay for not showing courage and humility and listening only to so-called friends who will only lend you an ear and speak soft words is that nothing will ever change, and you will dye with your problem unsolved.

We all tend to appreciate sympathetic listeners who seem to understand our predicaments. There are endless sympathetic listeners around but, somehow, their advice never seems to make any difference in changing our bad habits. Consider that and develop COURAGE and HUMILITY. Stop sparing your ego! There lies the only "miracle solution."

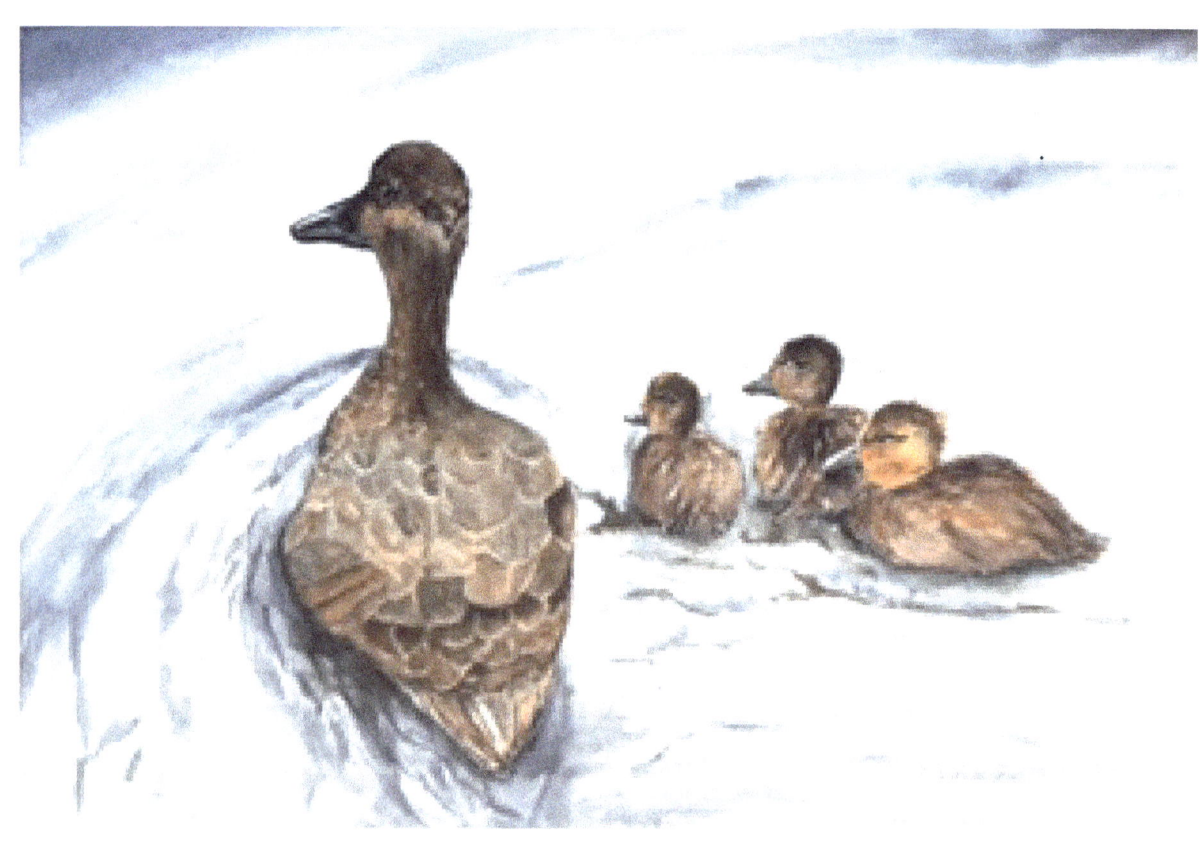

Our Belief System Dictates Whom We Will Attract or Be Attracted to /
I Don't Want to Get Hurt, So I Will Not Let Anybody In

Our Belief System Dictates Whom We Will Attract Or Be Attracted To

As we experience the hardships of life and are subjected to the various influences of our families and acquaintances, we develop our own set of beliefs to fit our personal nature. Thus, someone who tends to be easily disappointed may be attracted by soft-spoken and rather "neutral" personalities and will shy away from strong, challenging people. A person of overbearing character may be attracted by a submissive type. A selfless individual may be drawn to poor or needy people, etc. And, due to everyone's individual experience of life, such combinations are varied, each leading to the development of a personal set of beliefs. In this merry-go-round, total confusion reigns; thus, unless one keeps a very humble and open attitude, it becomes easy to say "I don't agree with you" since there is no balance in such a chaos and the ego takes over readily.

I Don't Want to Get Hurt, So I Will Not Let Anybody In

A fairly sure way not to get profoundly hurt in your feelings by others is simply to avoid developing close relationships, especially intimate ones. But for many, this may not be the best solution. For, remember that if no one is allowed into your life, no one will be able to contribute to it either. Our greatest deceptions do come from other human beings; but so do our greatest joys. A pet such as a dog can, indeed, be a safe choice since it will provide you with steadfast companionship. But while avoiding a possible roller coaster of emotions, you will also bypass the greatest joys life has to offer. Let me stress that humankind encompasses a bit of everything, from the worst to the best… and chances are that if your ultimate goal is to become the best person you can be, it follows that you will attract very good people as well.

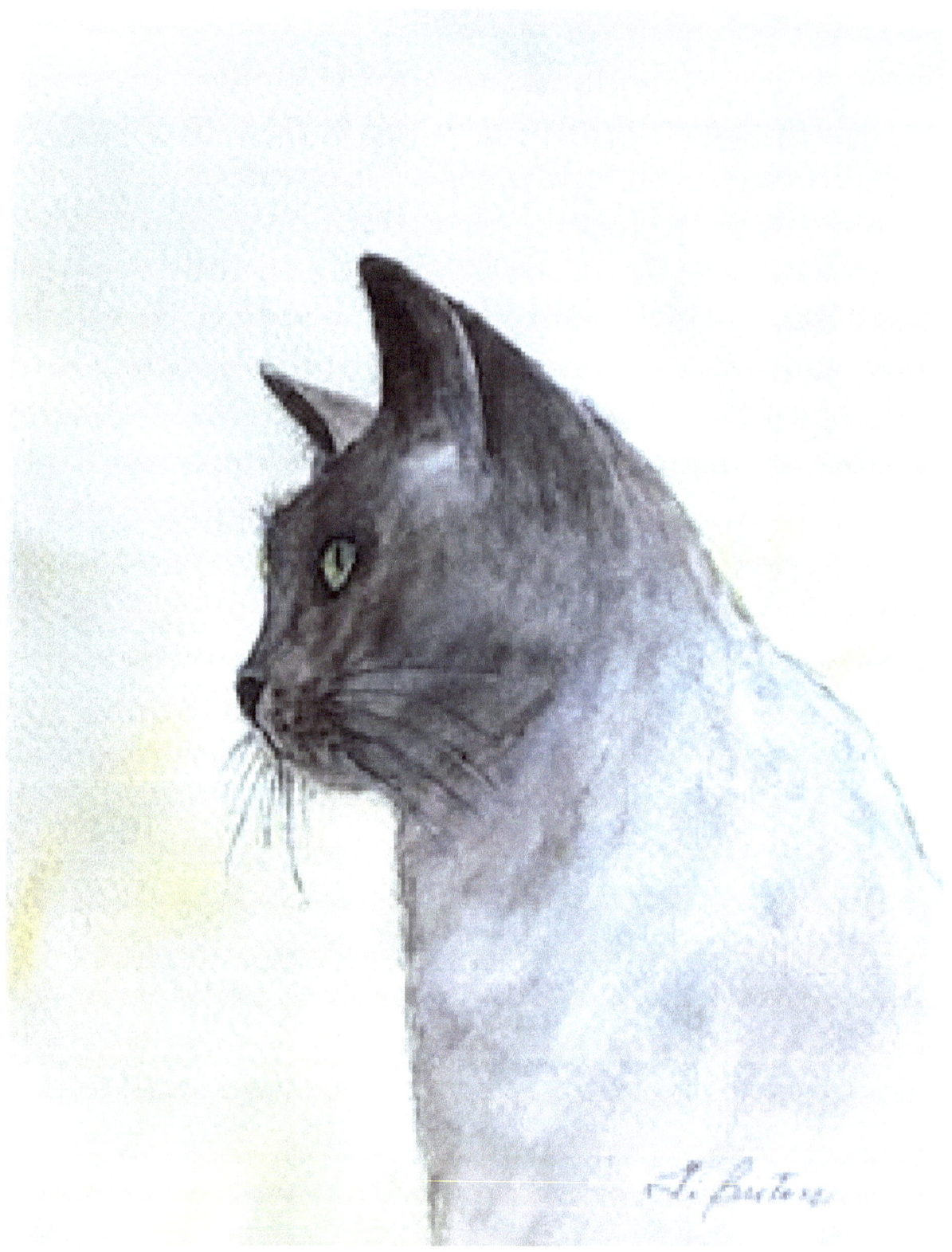

False Modesty and the Inability to Say Things as We See Them

So far in this book, we have alluded several times to the idea of harmonizing so-called opposites so as to evolve spiritually. Of course, there is cold and hot, tiny and immense, dark and light, stingy and generous, soft and hard, gentle and violent, mean and kind... should I go on with the list?

This ego of ours which we have to tame constantly gets in the way. It says: "I'm right and your wrong," "I disagree with you," etc. Meanwhile, our spiritual being that has great trouble revealing itself through such hopeless upheaval is trying in a whisper to remind us that we are following a dead-end street. As a result, instead of mending our ways, we resort to false modesty. A few individuals who have succeeded in silencing this inner spiritual voice do brag unhampered about their accomplishments, their intelligence, and their realizations. But for most, the faint little voice tells them that it is wrong to do so. Unfortunately, instead of leaving this dead-end trail of confrontation, they counteract by simply resorting to false modesty. Harmonizing opposites would mean being able to openly and honestly talk about both your flaws AND your qualities when necessary (no boasting involved). Just describe reality as you perceive it. Did you ever try to ask someone who is passionate about skiing, for instance, if he or she is an excellent skier? Chances are that the answer you will get is: "Not so bad." Being aware that it is not a good idea to brag, we diminish our accomplishments instead of reaching a balance between our flaws and qualities. It would then seem that false modesty is also anchored in ego considerations rather than in the truth as we perceive it.

Having spent some fifty-five years of my life teaching languages, I will not hesitate to tell you that I became an expert over the years in developing techniques to better convey my knowledge to my students (which includes teaching self-defence martial arts). Yet, if you ask me how well I perform when it comes to mathematics, I will readily and unambiguously confess that I manage poorly in this regard. My close friends, who almost know me inside out, will know that I am neither basking in "self-appreciation" nor bathing in self-depreciation, but simply saying the truth as I perceive it. But I will let you guess what the average Joe Blow would think if he heard me say that I am an expert teacher.

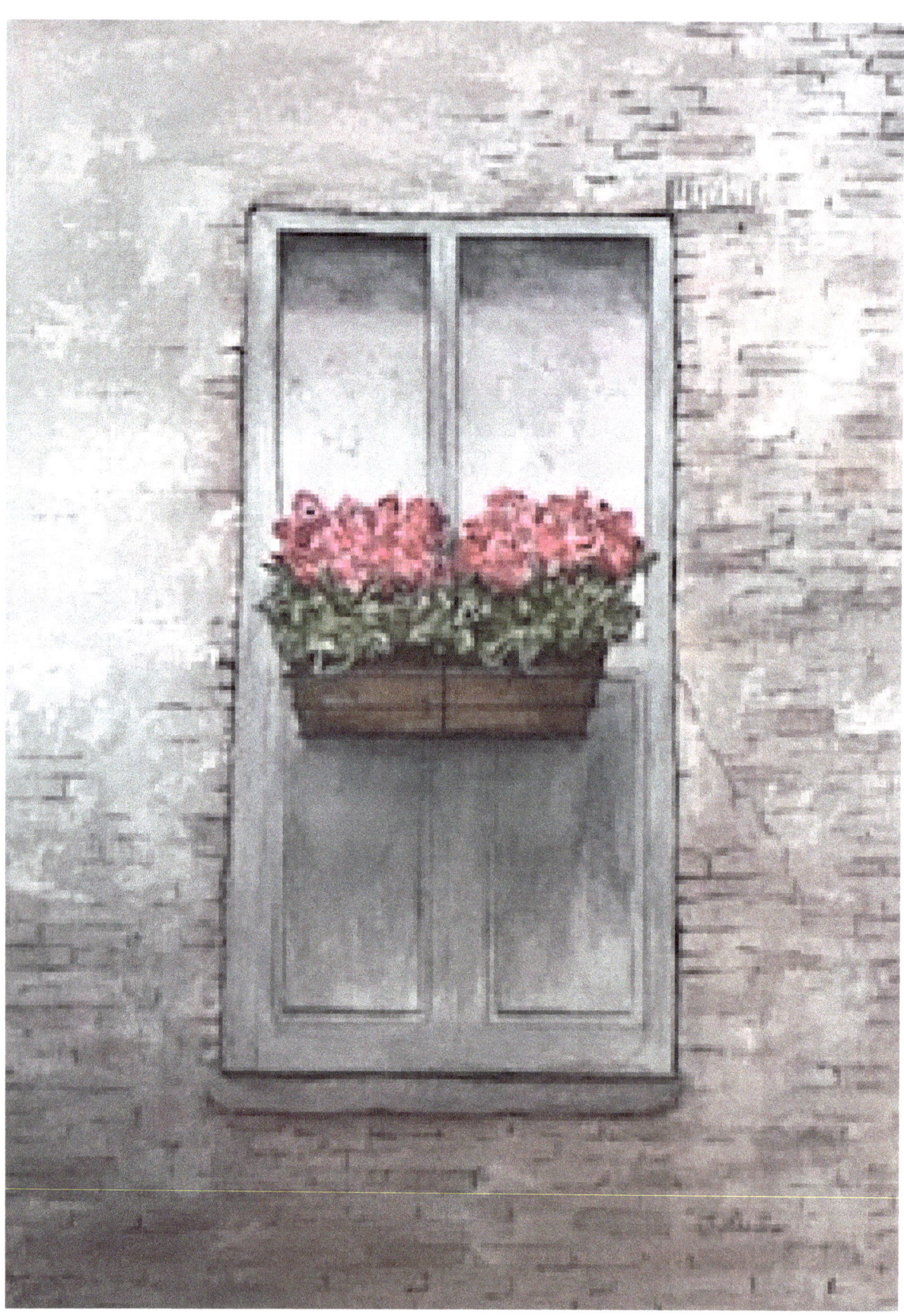

Time And Timelessness

We are so used to living with the clock and measuring our daily activities in terms of seconds, minutes, hours, days, months, years, etc. that we easily lose track of the timeless dimension of the universe and everything in it. For instance, the **observable** universe is 94 billion light years across. A single light year covers 9.4607×10^{12} km which is almost 6 trillion miles. This is what we can actually observe; but given the proper conditions, who knows what we would find beyond. According to NASA, "This suggests that the universe is infinite in extent; however, since the universe has a finite age, we can only observe a finite volume of the universe." Now think for a moment… as you and I are busy writing or reading these lines within a limited time frame, the world we live in is basically timeless for all intents and purposes. In the 18th century, Antoine Laurent Lavoisier (who is the father of modern chemistry according to some) told us that «nothing is lost, and nothing is created» but that everything is **transformed**.

Talking about what we can observe, simply look at the animal kingdom. I know that some species have highly sophisticated means of communication, such as whales. These animals travel in pods using different noises to communicate with each other namely clicks, pulsed calls and whistles to help them navigate, identify their physical surroundings or to socialize. Now, compare this with the more than 7000 languages spoken around the world. For that matter, just think of your own English, French, German, or Spanish language to name a few and how beautifully complex they are to allow human beings to express refined ideas, create highly advanced technologies, develop beautiful poetry, and permit innumerable other tasks way beyond our daily necessities for survival. But consider also that only our human species can create sophisticated weapons to wage wars and destroy other people.

As I am presently reading "***Das menschliche Gehirn, Eine Gebrauchsanweisung***", a German translation of American author John J. Ratey, I can only marvel at the design of our brain, this dynamic organ created by nature through evolution. But beyond our *physical brain*, we are the only species on earth that has a truly spiritual component. While wild animals mostly fight and kill for their survival, the ego in human beings too often veils our spiritual component which leads to the domination and destruction of others, in total opposition to our wonderful potential for harmonious creation. Descartes used to say "Cogito, ergo sum" or "I think, therefore I am". But it took a few centuries for thinkers to understand that ego (the "I" in "I think" or "I am") is not to be confused with our spiritual potential.

Again, should we not tame the ego and learn to harmonize opposites such as "time" and "timelessness" by developing our awareness of this timeless component which is our spiritual potential instead of staying at this time-constricted level of the ego? While our ego is directly associated with our earthly identity regarding our past and our future (since it is concerned with where our human brain has led us and will lead until we die), our spiritual identity focusses on the present moment and is not concerned with our past or future feats. Some activities concentrate by definition on the present moment, whether we are painting, composing a piece of music, admiring a beautiful sunset, smelling the perfume of a flower, writing a piece of poetry, etc. They are then partaking in our spiritual potential which is timeless and has no regrets about the past nor fear of what lies ahead.

Here is a very concrete overview of what the ego says, using some everyday examples:

1. I think that… (opinion);
2. I don't agree with…(conflict);
3. I don't give a damn about… (division/indifference);
4. I'm afraid this will not work… (apprehension);
5. I wish I could… (uncertainty/inability);
6. Who does he think he is telling me that… (pride);
7. I don't believe this will work… (defeatism);
8. I shouldn't have trusted her… (regret);
9. I am totally infatuated with her… (blindesness);
10. Who cares what happens to him… (heartlessness);
11. He's a criminal and we should have no mercy… (self-righteousness);
12. I don't trust men anymore… (fear);
13. They can all go to hell… (anger);
14. She says that because she's jealous… (envy/interpretation);
15. I wouldn't give such people the time of day (contempt);
16. Etc.

If you have not found much positive in what precedes… I don't blame you! The ego is a very poor "adviser". Add to this the fact that our brain is constantly busy pushing ideas through our minds, and you have the perfect recipe for remaining detached from (or should I say, "unaware" of) your spiritual being. In other words, staying at that level will ensure that you live your material life in a permanent illusion since your spirit is the real you. It is timeless and can participate directly in the creative process of the universe. This is where you get in touch with universal love and beauty. So then, you might ask why, as children, we in fact gradually move away from the simplicity and spontaneity we share with the animal kingdom and slowly but surely develop our ego (which, by the way, all animal species don't seem to have). There lies this apparent contradiction. Evolution has slowly led us to become "thinkable" beings, free to choose between so-called opposites of good/bad, weak/strong, etc. as previously stated in a former chapter. We have to reconcile these elements and the best way to do so is by creating space for contemplation in our present lives. Relearn to act as a child and take time to "stop and smell the roses". Take time to be in awe before the beautiful spectacle of the sun setting on the ocean waters, etc. Learn to interpret the challenges of life as opportunities to grow instead of wallowing in self-pity. Appreciate what you have instead of focussing on what you lost or don't have.

Here is a concrete overview of some of the ways you can get closer to your spiritual, eternal being:

1. Grow a garden and admire life as it takes form in various ways from tiny seeds.
2. Listen to great musical creations with a total focus on the vibrations and notes and their harmonious combinations.
3. Participate in a physical activity, not to compete but rather to get in touch with others and your inner self. Traditional, non-competitive ju-jitsu such as **Bouei-Michi-Ryu** is a good example of this.
4. Go for walks regularly and train your mind to focus on your breathing and on anything you find beautiful such as trees, flowers, birds and their songs, etc.
5. Take up a hobby such as painting, playing a musical instrument and so forth, where all your attention is required to perform the task.
6. Make room in your life for meditative moments.
7. When going through "tough times," learn to see what positive lessons you can derive from that and be grateful for this opportunity to grow.
8. Learn to appreciate what you have instead of focussing on what you don't have.
9. Set yourself a goal of becoming the best human being you can be.
10. Learn to truly listen to what others have to say.
11. Learn to care for the plight of others who, for instance, live in war-ravaged countries.
12. Learn to give to and share with those less fortunate.
13. Learn to love your "so-called enemies," and those you may initially have found "unlovable."
14. Learn to harmonize "so-called opposites;" for example, being strong, skilled, and determined to fight, physically or otherwise, to save lives and yet, being sensitive and forgiving when necessary.
15. Keep reminding yourself that it is easy to love "lovable" people, but that loving those who might seem despicable is an absolute necessity to make this world a better place to live.
16. Etc.

All of the above should help you live this time-constricted life in a timeless perspective, as previously stated, since it brings you in touch with your eternal, spiritual entity.

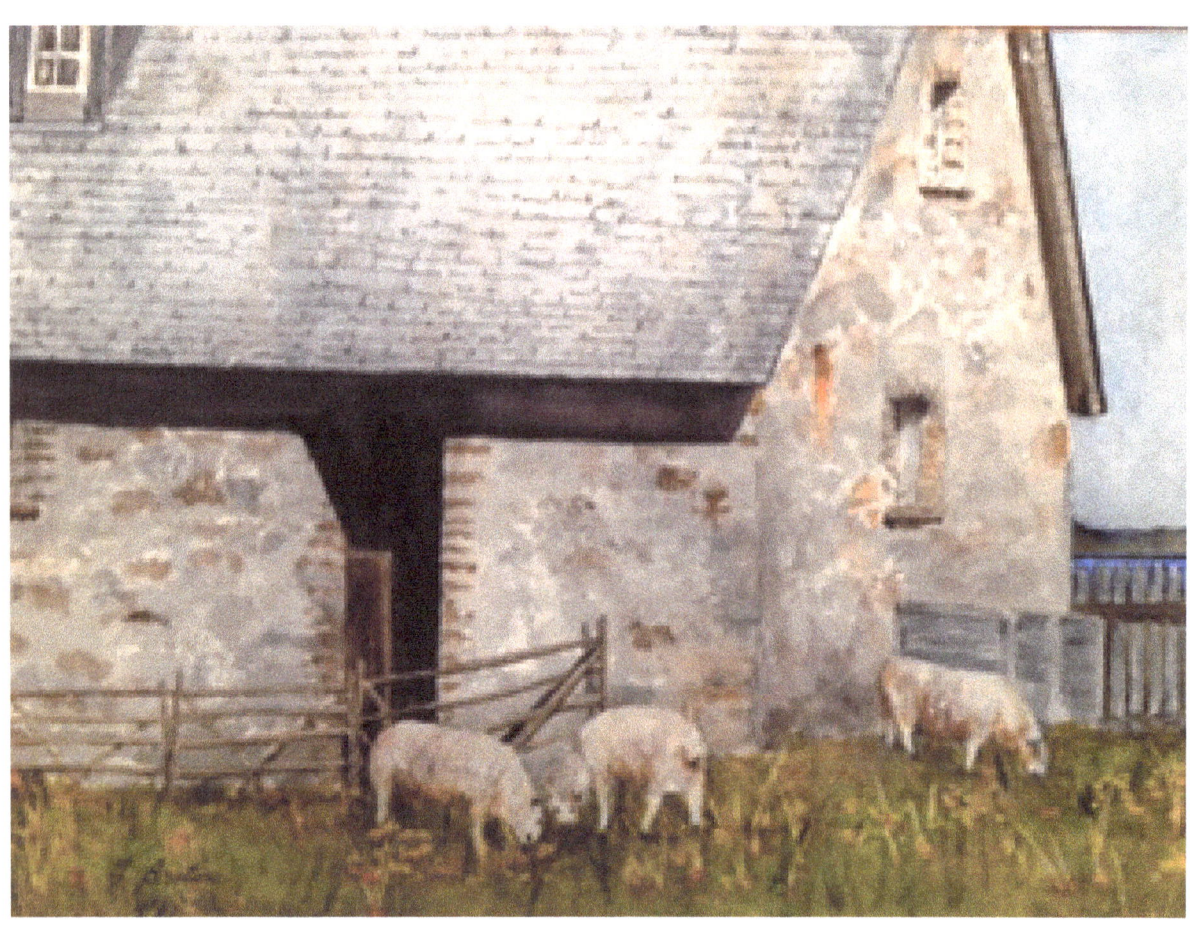

Getting Used to Miracles

Natural Miracles

Compared with other planets surrounding the earth, the generous nature around us is absolutely astounding and full of miracles. There is not only an infinity of colours, fragrances, and so on for us to enjoy, but also a great variety of plants and animals. Needless to say that humans also have tremendous potential overall, as can be seen by our immense creative abilities. But contrary to the sure way that balance is constantly re-established in the natural world, humans have difficulty finding balance and can be very destructive as well. Could it be that we easily lose track of the miracle of life and get used too quickly to our surroundings? Science is indeed more and more capable of devising tools and technologies to analyse complex organs such as the brain; but we are still leagues away from explaining how all of this came about. Some find solace in referring to Darwin's theory of evolution; however, this theory explains very little if only that the various vegetable and animal species on earth evolved over millions of years. This is far more an observation than a true explanation. Yet, as soon as one delves into the present moment and connects with all of these "unexplainable" manifestations through our spiritual ability (which is eternal), everything becomes clear, and we are at peace with all of creation. It is so easy to let our mind become entangled in familiar, everyday tasks that we readily forget the miracle of life.

Religious Miracles

Many religions throughout history have perceived unexplainable events as divine miracles, particularly as it relates to sudden physical healings. I was raised in a catholic family and remember that, as a child, I was intrigued by the yearly visits of a priest from the archdiocese, coming to confirm the miraculous healing of my mother so as to eventually be able to canonize Brother André with the many similar cases that had allowed crippled or terminally ill people to walk away miraculously healed after having prayed before his shrine at the St-Joseph Oratory in Montreal. Having personally no attachment to any particular religion (although I definitely consider myself a spiritual being), I tend to think that the miracle rather lies in the fact that we possess still unexplained self-healing capabilities.

What some health care workers sometimes describe in a somewhat negative way as the placebo effect, I view as the yet-to-be-harnessed capability of humans to heal themselves, given the right circumstances. For those not too familiar with the term "placebo", I might simply say that it refers to a given medication that contains no active substances capable of restoring health and yet, when given to the patient as real medication, causes healing in the subject involved. We should rather be in awe before the self-healing capabilities of our body. For instance, just think of how your skin or flesh can heal itself after being scratched or burnt. We expect this to happen automatically in everyday life and tend to easily forget that such self-healing capabilities are in themselves somewhat "miraculous".

> Beauty is in the eye of the beholder
> *Old Proverb*

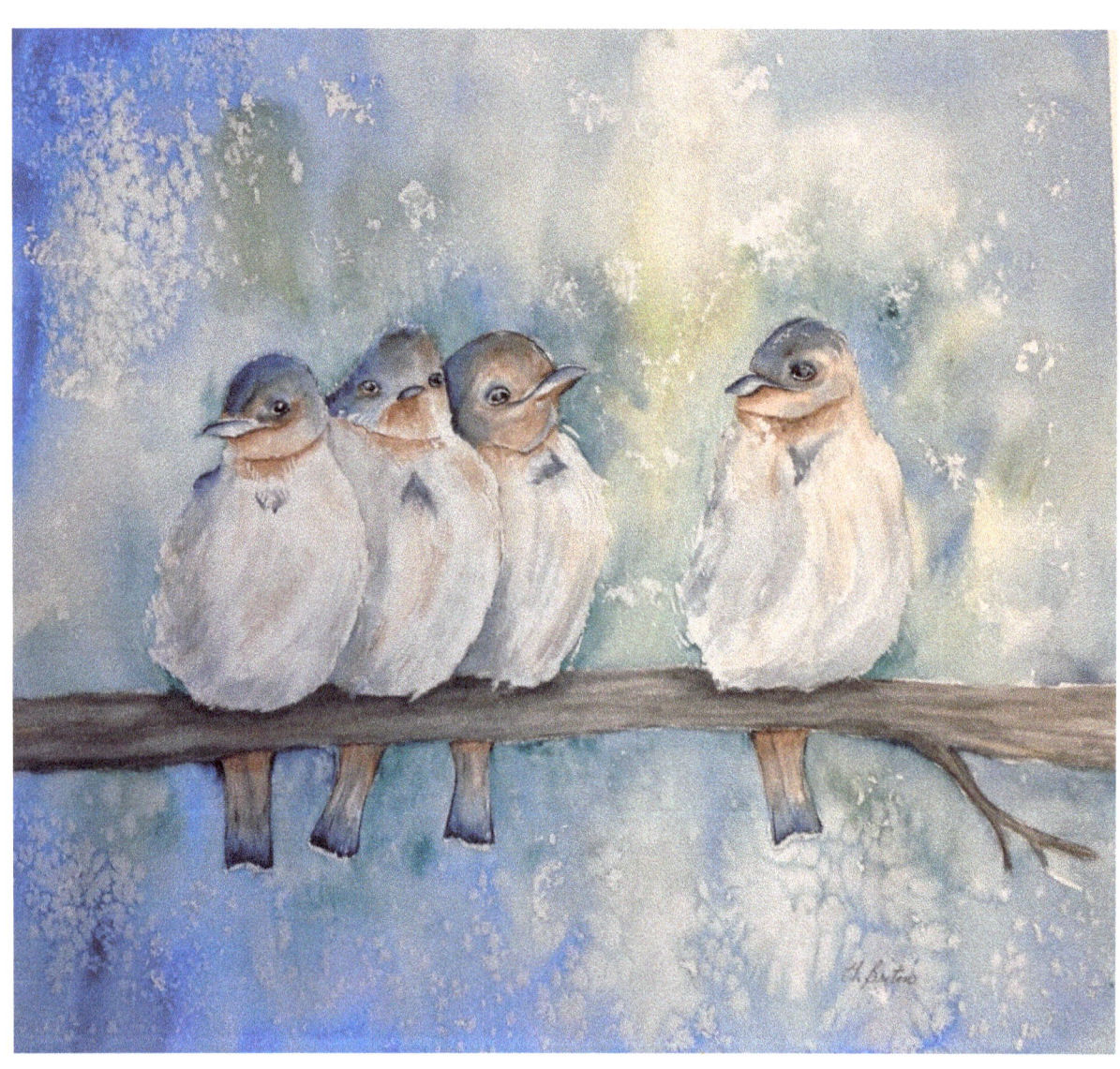

How Can We Be Sure That There Is Life After Death?

Is that question useful?

We have already seen that the universe we live in right now is boundless and that the notion of time is also relative. Those are not beliefs but rather, scientifically proven facts. As far back as we can go in the history of mankind, people's basic and natural need for certainty has led humans to look for signs of assurance that there is life after death. Innumerable religions were based on that belief. According to Chaplain Darrell W. Wood, "Across the eons of human history, the search for immortality and life after death has been a universal quest in religious faith and practice. Egyptian pyramids were built as tombs for the pharaohs and their consorts during the Old and Middle Kingdom as an expression of belief in the structure to be a means to immortality and a portal to the afterlife."

It stands to reason that as soon as the human species evolved beyond the animal kingdom (whose soul and basic need is that of survival), and became "aware" of its own existence, the question of survival beyond our material form came into play. This not only illustrates our need for certainty but also coincides with our natural need to progress and grow, as well as the need to contribute to society (or should we say, to humanity.) We don't need to spend a lifetime in meditation to get in touch with our spirituality, but it certainly helps if we develop the habit of saving moments in our daily routine for "meditative space" i.e., for moments when we stop regretting the past or worrying about the future and focus on the present moment to stop this constant flow of ideas that crowd our mind and leave little space for appreciating the beauties of creation and our direct connection to the divine. To say it in a different way, if we stop listening to this ego of ours that wants us to affirm our superiority over other people because we are supposedly richer, taller, more intelligent, more handsome, more skillful, etc., and simply listen to our need to contribute instead of dominating, then our chances of appreciating the beauty of creation increases accordingly. What precedes leads us back to this principle of harmonizing opposites to bloom as entities. In this case, such opposites are, on the one hand, the need to dominate (compete) and on the other hand, the need to contribute (serve). Hence the quasi-irrelevance of the question "How can we be sure that there is life after death?" I would rather suggest getting in touch, at various moments, with the spiritual component of our life instead of letting our mind be submerged non-stop with earthly preoccupations. How about living your **immortal spirituality** right now?

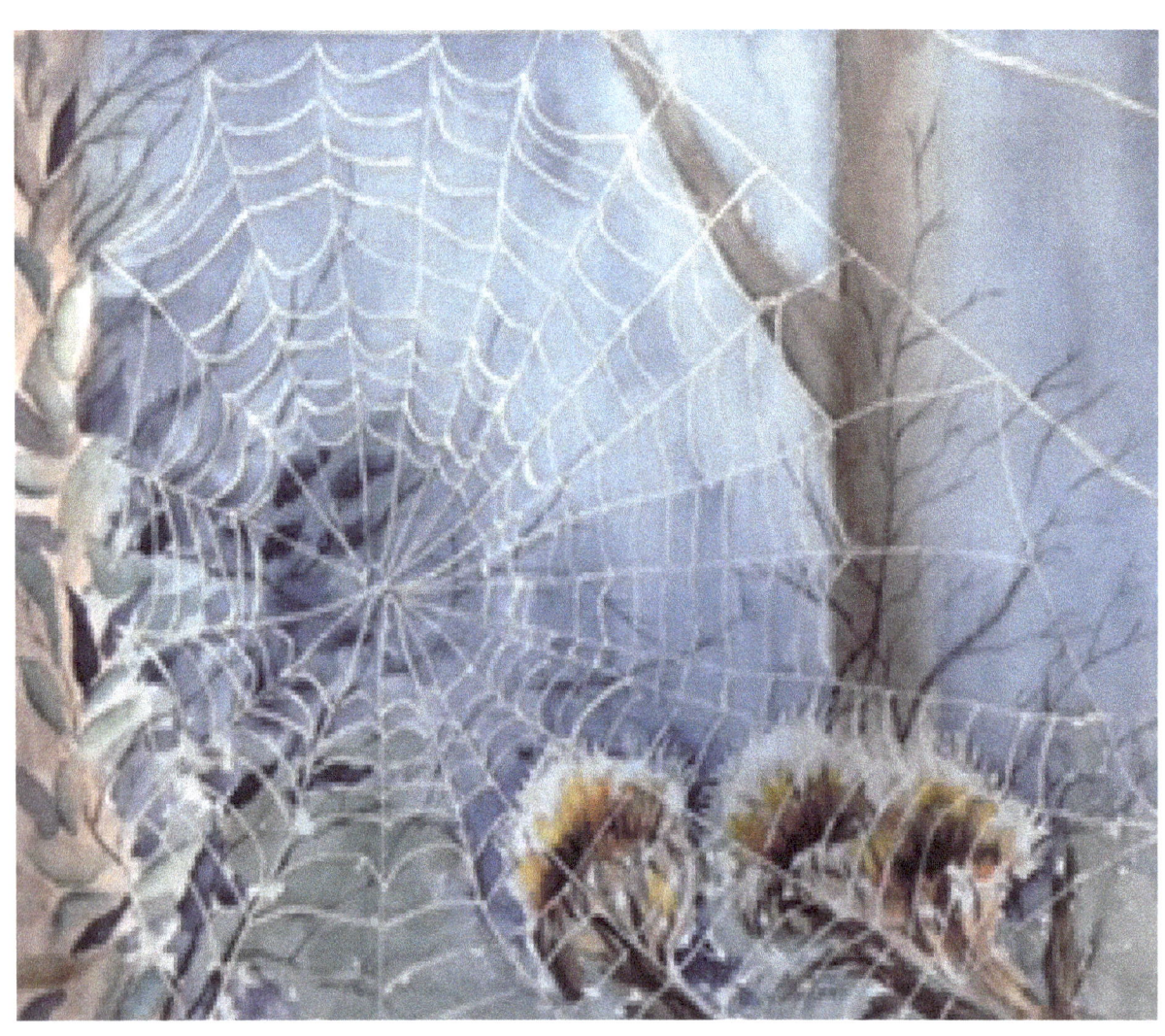

Being Grateful

Being Grateful (What Is the Outcome of Being Grateful?)

The very first advantage of being grateful that comes to mind is that it keeps you in a positive mood. Let us look at the process of getting old, for instance, since I am almost an expert in that area at my age. As you advance in age, your energy level tends to somewhat decrease. Instead of dwelling on all the activities you could do at a younger age and settling for a sedentary, inactive life, why not learn from that and be grateful for everything else you have? Instead of giving up on yourself, learn how to maximize the level of energy you still have to perform the activities still within your reach. For instance, go for long and healthy walks, develop a simple routine to exercise your arms, your back, etc. Soon, these habits will become part of you and will re-energize you. One of the types of energies still within reach is that of being "passionate" about your friendships, the experience you have acquired over the years, etc. The more grateful you are, the more passionate you will be. This will attract others like a real magnet, which will put you in a position to contribute to their well-being. For, being grateful for the opportunity to share and contribute is one of the best gifts that life has in store for you.

When you are grateful, fear disappears, and abundance appears.
Anthony Robbins

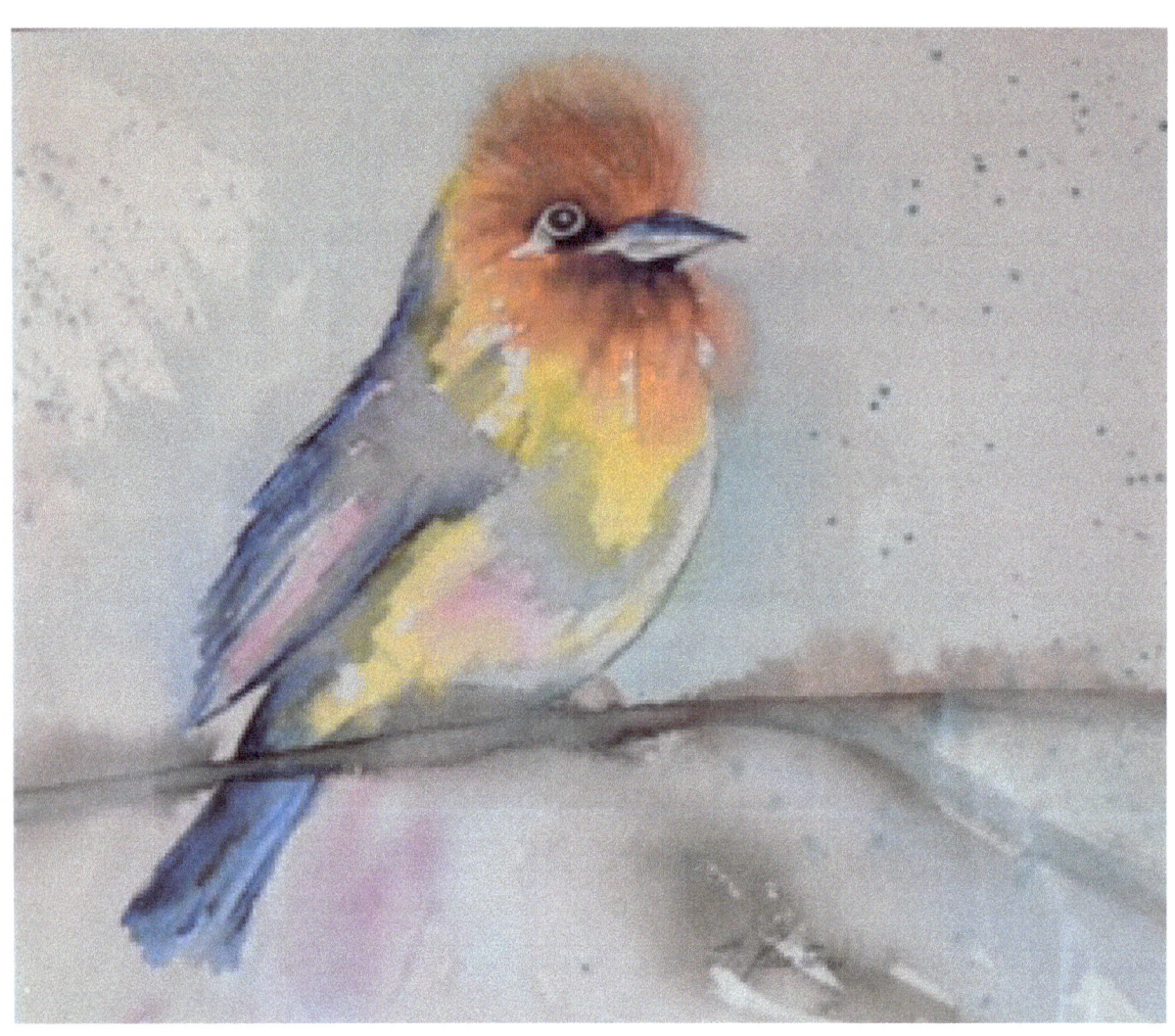

Is Giving Superior to Receiving?

If you interpret this question from a religious angle, chances are that your answer will be "yes". Religions tend to perceive such notions from a moral point of view. Thus, "giving" is morally "good" while "receiving" has no such virtue. But "good" and "bad" are opposite perceptions which lead us directly to the concept of "ego". If I give of my time or my money, etc., the ensuing conclusion is that I am a good person, while keeping it all to myself should make me an egoistical individual. (Notice the connection between "ego" and "egoistical".) Knowing how to "receive" (gifts, ideas, a helping hand, etc.) gracefully from others may also have its merits and opens doors to a much smoother and effortless development. Be it as it may, there may be a different way to approach this subject.

As you grow spiritually by taking time off from the everyday humdrum and by delving into your inner self, you should gradually discover that you are part of a whole... part and parcel of the immensity of the universe. The tiniest parcel of our body encompasses both the intelligence and elements of creation. Such notions as "good" and "bad" then become if not irrelevant, at least "opposites to reconcile" since we each form part of a whole and are simply at different stages of development. Lions preying on a zebra are not bad; they simply follow their instinct to survive according to their rank in the evolution of the animal kingdom. A dictator is not bad; he simply acts in accordance with his degree of evolution in the human realm. This is not to say that we should submit and accept all the atrocities committed by belligerent leaders, but simply that we should move towards the other end of the spectrum, i.e., towards love and harmony and reach a balance between both. As previously stated in this book, *"the only things truly worth fighting for, it seems to me, are the protection of the gift of life and freedom of choice."*

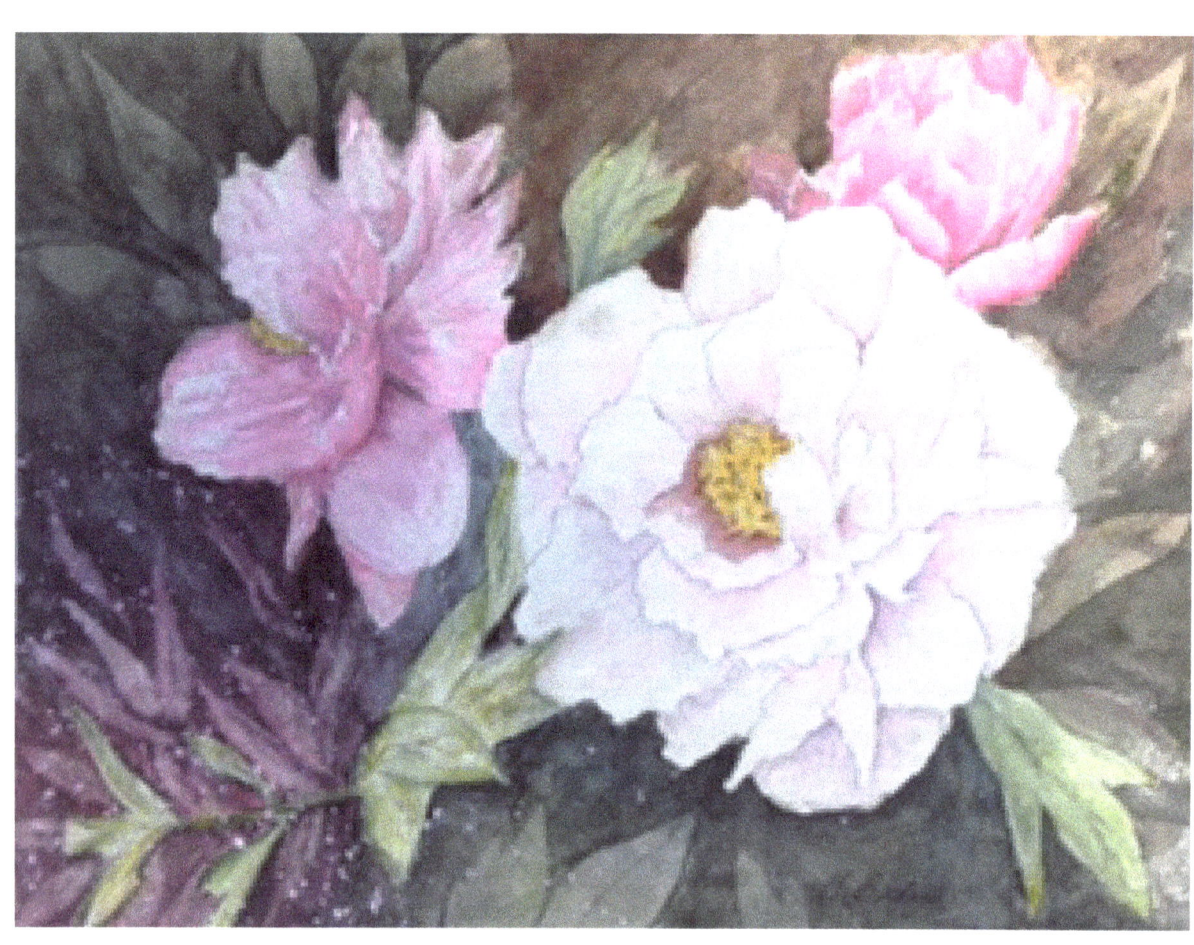

"Love," this overused word

One of the most overused words in our language is the noun or verb "love". If you look up the word in the Merriam-Webster dictionary, you will find definitions along the following lines for the noun:

- Strong affection for another arising out of kinship or personal ties – Example: maternal love for a child.
- Attraction based on sexual desire: affection and tenderness felt by lovers – Example: After all these years, they are still very much in love.
- Affection based on admiration, benevolence, or common interests – Example: love for his old schoolmates.
- An assurance of affection – Example: give her my love.
- Warm attachment, enthusiasm, or devotion – Example: love of the sea.
- The object of attachment, devotion, or admiration – Example: baseball was his first love.
- A beloved person: DARLING – Often used as a term of endearment.
- (British) —used as an informal term of address.
- Unselfish loyal and benevolent concern for the good of another: such as the fatherly concern of God for humankind or brotherly concern for others.
- A person's adoration of God.
- A god (such as Cupid or Eros) or personification of love.
- An amorous episode: LOVE AFFAIR.
- The sexual embrace: COPULATION.

…And we could go on and on with such definitions or examples.

Although it is not my intent to redefine the word itself, I think we would have advantage in making the following three main distinctions:

- Strong attachment to an object, an activity, etc.
- Sexual attraction for another person.
- Deep and profound concern for the well-being of another human being.

With such distinctions, we might better understand such expressions as the following ones, instead of treating them as having equal value:

- I love this car/my job/etc. (attachment);
- to fall in love (infatuation) / to make love (sexual encounter).
- …as opposed to giving of oneself for the benefit and wellbeing of someone else without expecting anything in return (love in the truest sense).

For indeed, one might wonder what does in fact happen when one **falls in love**.

1. Do we fill a gap after having felt lonely for some time?
2. Do we truly see the person as he/she is or are we looking at a reflection of our own desires, since we have no history with this person and may simply be blinded by the "newness" of it all?

Note: The reasons one "falls in love" are as varied as the list of "qualities" mentioned by those looking for a partner in a dating agency. Example: I'm looking for a tall/thin/young/handsome/good looking partner who practices sports, etc. If there is a match, then Bingo! …one may fall in love.

No judgment intended, but I personally prefer partners who "grow in love" as years go by. For, growing in love not only implies developing attachment but also, learning to truly care for the person sharing our life.

Why is it that, contrary to the animal kingdom, we find in humans contradictory aspirations such as, on the one hand, the need to help and contribute, but on the other hand, the desire to take advantage of others and exploit them? Somebody gets attacked by hoodlums in broad daylight as you are walking by. What will you do? Will you come to the rescue of this individual? A few might come to the assistance of the victim risking their own lives in the process. Many won't even bother to call 911 for assistance, being too busy "watching the show" and even if the risk of making such a call is limited. Another minority might even wait to see if they cannot further take advantage of the unconscious victim, by stealing whatever could still be of value such as a neckless, etc. assuming that there are no longer any witness around. We have all heard of helpless victims of a calamity (hurricane, flood, etc.) being victimized a second time by rogues looting the debris of their homes.

In nature, a vulture would readily pick at an animal's lame body left to dye. It would have no sense of guilt or regrets in doing so. But on the other hand, some species might risk their own lives to protect the most vulnerable members of their herd or flock. Many of us follow this animal instinct. But why is it that, some humans have a calling to love others (strangers) unconditionally. We have seen this calling in rare, illuminated prophets who were even prepared to give up their lives for the well-being of others… Jesus-Christ, Gandhi, etc.

Of the preceding paragraphs, I would venture to make the following remarks:

Humans have indeed a spiritual calling to develop universal love, instead of simply acting instinctively like the animal kingdom. This gradual awakening is called "satori" in Japanese Buddhism and should eventually lead to "nirvana".

> Love is "the will to extend one's self for the purpose of nurturing one's own or another's spiritual growth."
>
> *M. Scott Peck, M.D.*

Gilberte Breton's
Artistic Career

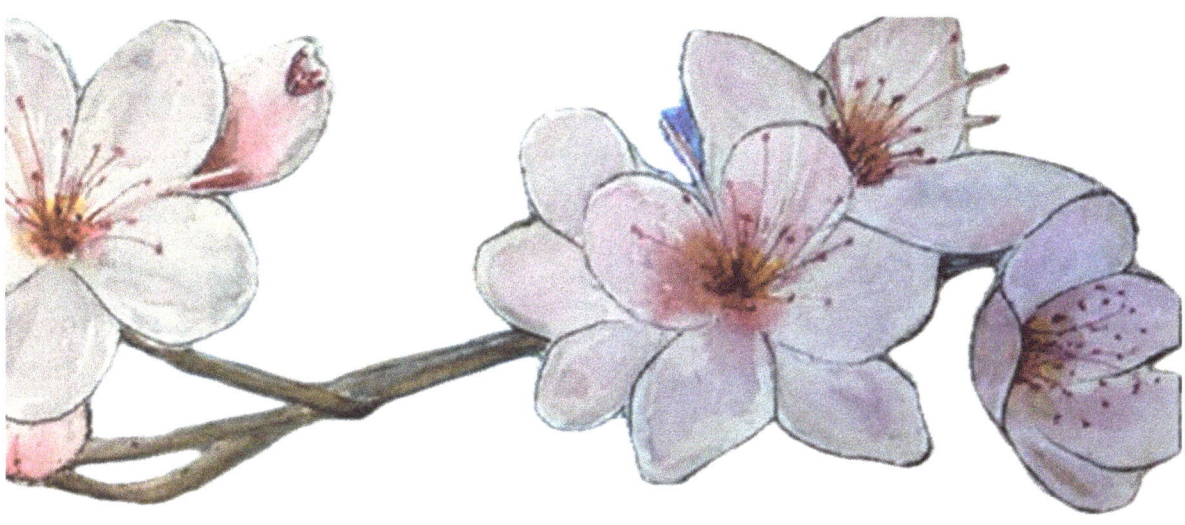

Throughout the various stages of her life, Gilberte has always shown great interest in anything of an artistic nature, whether it be knitting, sewing, cooking, drawing and of course, painting. No sooner had she retired that she fulfilled her life-long dream and registered in watercolour classes. Her first teacher was Suzanne Lemieux who taught her the basics related to this medium. Then came Madeleine Laberge with whom she perfected her technique. Meanwhile, she joined a workgroup of watercolourists. For the last 16 years, she has been blissfully devoting a full day per week to her passion. Part of her production was exhibited on numerous occasions in various artistic events.